I0791074

Keto Way of Life:

Ketogenic Plans For a Healthier Life

Teresa Fikes

&

Georgann R.Fohner

ISBN: 9781670885593
Imprint: Independently published

Please note the information contained within this document is for educational and entertainment purposes only. Every attempt has been made to provide accurate, up to date, and reliable complete information. No warranties of any kind are expressed or implied. Readers acknowledge that the author is not engaged in the rendering of legal, financial, medical, or professional advice.

By reading this document, the reader agrees that under no circumstances are we responsible for any losses, direct or indirect, which are incurred as a result of the use of the information contained within this document, including, but not limited to, —errors, omissions, or inaccuracies.

Table Of Contents

Introduction

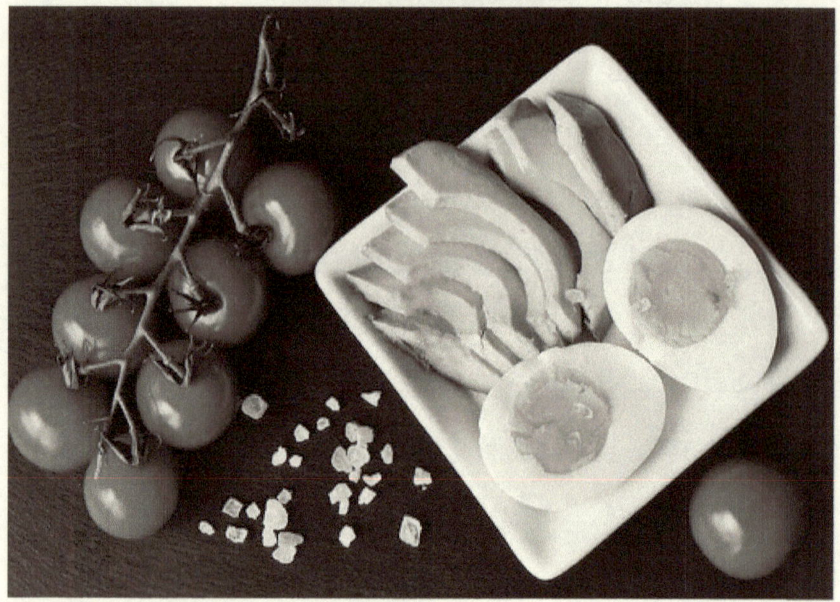

A ketogenic diet is so much more than just a "diet". The ketogenic diet is actually a lifestyle change. It is about learning how to eat all over again, the ketogenic lifestyle is about learning how to transform the way we look at and move toward a new method of eating.

 The principle idea behind being on a ketogenic diet is for you to create a state known as "Ketosis" for your body to enter into. The best part about being on the Keto diet is that there are no expensive products to purchase. You will discover that everything about the Keto diet is inexpensive, with everyday items you purchase at your local supermarket. No expensive, unknown supplements that are difficult to find are required on the Keto diet.

You will discover, as you read each section of this ebook the Ketogenic Lifestyle is much more than a diet. You will learn how to live the Ketogenic way of life, and how simple it will be to learn how to eat healthy, how to lose that unwanted weight and how to finally keep it off. All of this will be accomplished once you have learned that a Ketogenic Lifestyle is like no other "diet" you have ever tried. So read on, my dear reader, and learn how to start creating a more healthy lifestyle in which you will begin to look and feel the best you have ever felt.

I would like to thank you in advance, my dear reader, for taking the time to purchase the book *"Keto Lifestyle: Ketogenic to a Healthier, Longer Life."* Some interesting points this book will cover involve the following:

- What is a Ketogenic diet?
- The different types of Ketogenic diets there are
- How do you deal with the effects of the "Keto Flu"?
- How to know when you have reached "ketosis"
- Are there any hazards to being on a Keto diet?
- Plus, many more interesting information about living a Ketogenic life

Here's an inescapable fact: you will need to read this ebook in its entirety in order to learn how to live this new lifestyle and receive all the advantages and benefits of living a Ketogenic Lifestyle.

So now that you know you are about to embark on a brand new healthy lifestyle, are you ready to learn more? As you read each chapter and learn how easy it is to create this new healthy lifestyle, there will be only one question you will have for yourself and that question will be: "Where has this diet and lifestyle been all your life and why did it take so long to finally learn about it?"

Chapter 1
"What Is a Ketogenic Diet?"

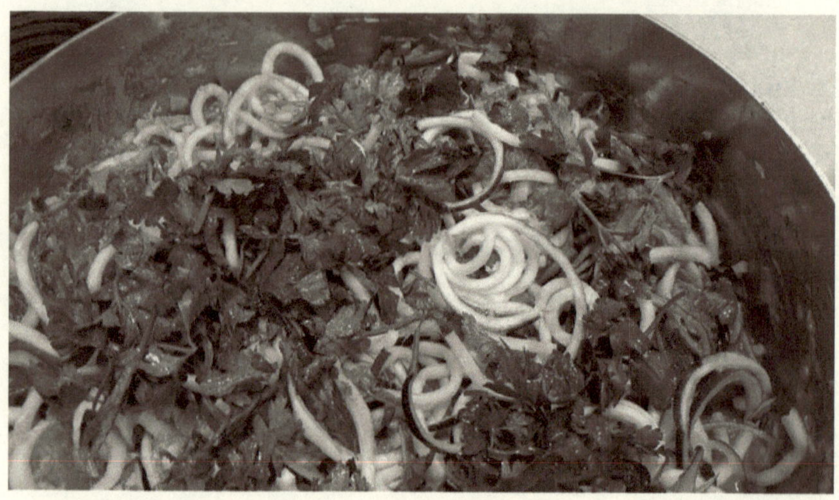

This diet known as the "ketogenic diet" is a diet that is a high-fat, a diet that has a sufficient amount of protein, and reduced carbohydrates. The ketogenic diet gained its popularity by being one of the primary methods that medical personnel uses to treat hard-to-control epilepsy in children. The way the keto diet works is to influence the body about how to convert fat grams instead of carbohydrates into a source of energy. Typically carbohydrates are transformed into glucose which is vital for proper brain operation. When on the keto diet, there are very little carbohydrates available; therefore, the liver starts to work on changing the fat into fatty acids and ketone bodies. These ketone bodies can then go through to the brain and exchange the glucose into a source of energy. When the body enters into a state of "ketosis" which is created by the increased quantity of ketone bodies within the blood, it then results in a decrease in the number of epileptic seizures. When children and young adults who have epileptic seizures go on a ketogenic diet at least half of them have found their seizures have been reduced by at least 50 percent.

A ketogenic diet is similar to the Atkins diet in that both are low-carbohydrate diets. The basic principle of a keto diet is for the person to derive more calories from protein and fat they consume and to get fewer calories from carbohydrates. When beginning a ketogenic regimine, you will first reduce caloric intake and carbohydrates from foods such as sugar, soda, pastries, and white bread. These types of foods are easily digested and high in carbohydrates.

The way the keto diet works is that when consuming fewer than 50 carbohydrates daily the body will begin to run low on fuel (also known as one's blood sugar); when this happens, the body is forced to start using protein and fat as its energy source. This is a process called ketosis. It usually takes about three to four days to reach the state of ketosis, once you reach ketosis you will begin to start losing weight.

When looking for a guideline to follow for a diet, the following list are what the typical person's body requires to lose weight efficiently:

- 60 to 75 percent of calories contain fat
- 15 to 30 percent are calories that contain protein
- 5 to 10 percent of the calories are carbohydrates

In order to achieve these guidelines while dieting it is a good idea to keep carb levels at about 20 to no more than 50 daily. It takes the body anywhere from two to seven days to delete all the carbohydrates that were once in the blood and to allow your body to enter into the ketosis state. This means that your body will begin to burn the fat and protein and convert it to energy; in which is the first step to your losing weight.

The ketogenic diet is also known as a "ketosis diet". What you are about to be doing when you begin the keto diet plan is you will be compelling your body to burn fat-- rather than carbohydrates-- and convert it to a source of energy that your body will be using.

Chapter 2
"Different Types of Keto Diets"

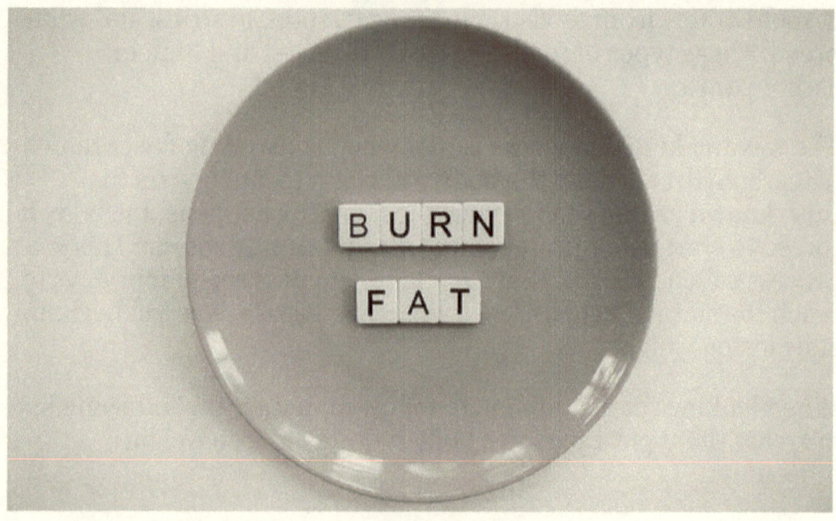

https://pixabay.com/photos/burn-fat-fat-burner-weight-loss-4235818/

There are four different types of Ketogenic diets:

- The Standard Ketogenic Diet
- The High Protein Ketogenic Diet
- The Cyclical Ketogenic Diet
- The Targeted Ketogenic Diet

Even though there are four different types of Keto diets, they all have the same approach-- and that is to aid the dieters in losing weight, burning fat, and creating a balance in the level of their blood sugar.

This chapter is going to go into each type of Keto Diet, what it involves and the type of person/dieter it will benefit the most.

If you are about to start Ketogenic diet, you are going to need to know about the different types of Ketogenic diets (there are more than one) the first keto diet we will discuss is the Standard Keto Diet (SKD).

The Standard Keto Diet

The Keto diet is an excellent way to rid yourself of the excess weight you have been working hard to lose. At the same time you can also enhance your current state of health by creating muscle, and make advancements in your physical fortitude.

The Standard Keto Diet (SKD) is a diet that is low in carbohydrates and high in fat. The amazing thing about the Keto diet is that you have always in the past heard that you should avoid fat grams at any cost when trying to lose weight. However, if you follow the Keto diet plan as it is prescribed to you, you are going to lose weight and learn how to live a healthier lifestyle in the process. By following the Standard Keto Diet plan, you will discover how to find a balance that fits your nutritional purpose.

Carbohydrates, protein, and fat are the primary focus when on the Standard Keto Diet plan. This diet is to limit carbohydrate intake, combined with a moderate amount of protein grams, and a whole lot of fat grams! By following this plan, you will be able to get your body into a state of ketosis, which is the way to lose weight. Cutting out carbohydrates from your daily diet forces your liver to create the ketones that are kept within the fat cells of your body and by eating a sufficient amount of protein while doing so will ensure your muscles remain intact.

When you want to stick to a diet and maintain a healthy weight loss it is imperative that you follow the guidelines of the Standard Keto Diet exactly as it is outlined. Below are the simple procedures in which have been set for your to follow:

- Avoid consuming an excessive amount of carbohydrates and protein; by doing so you will actually turn off the process of ketosis.
- Avoid consuming too much fat--this will create more body fat
- Ensure you eat an adequate amount of protein; a limited amount of protein will make you lose muscle mass
- As well, a limited amount of fats will sap your energy levels

The best way to lose weight in a healthy manner is to cut down on the amount of calories you consume daily by 10 to 15%. If you look at it from a nutritional standpoint it works out as the following formula:

* 40-60% fat
* 30-40% protein
* 10-20% carbohydrates

If it is possible to cut carbohydrates even lower, then by all means do so. Just ensure that when you are hungry you try to supplement your diet with fats and protein in order to meet your daily caloric goals.

The High Protein Keto Diet

The basic idea behind a high protein diet is that by limiting your carbohydrate intake you will force your body to burn the fat to produce energy. There are three types of high protein diets, Atkins, Dukan, and Keto. For the purpose of this book we will be discussing the Keto High Protein Diet.

The Keto diet is basically a high-protein, high-fat, low carbohydrate diet. You have to remember that if you eat too much protein and not enough fat you will prevent your body into getting into the ketosis state. So ensure yourself you are eating an adequate amount of fats.

The Cyclical Ketogenic Diet

The basis for the Cyclical Keto Diet is to alternate between the firm high-fat/low carbohydrate plan to allow for a little higher carbohydrate consumption.

When on a Cyclical Keto diet plan you follow the standard keto diet for five to six days and then increase your carbohydrate intake for the next one to two days. The idea behind this diet plan is to restore your body's natural glucose levels (which have been severely decreased). When you do this, you will leave the ketosis state which will permit your body to get all the advantages of a high carbohydrate diet for a brief period.

The Targeted Keto Diet (TKD)

The Targeted Keto Diet (TKD) is a diet in which you eat carbohydrates just before a workout, this approach offers the chance to enhance one's exercise routine. The TKD is designed for those athletes with stamina, weekend warriors, or for those who love an extensive exercise session.

If you feel totally run down and exhausted after a workout, the Targeted Keto Diet (TKD) may be just the thing for you. What you need is a high-carbohydrate diet to give you that extra energy. The TKD is just the diet a person who has issues keeping up with an intense workout needs. The extra carbohydrates in the TKD will aid you in keeping up your energy levels as you workout.

Chapter 3
"How Does a Ketogenic Diet Help you Lose Weight?"

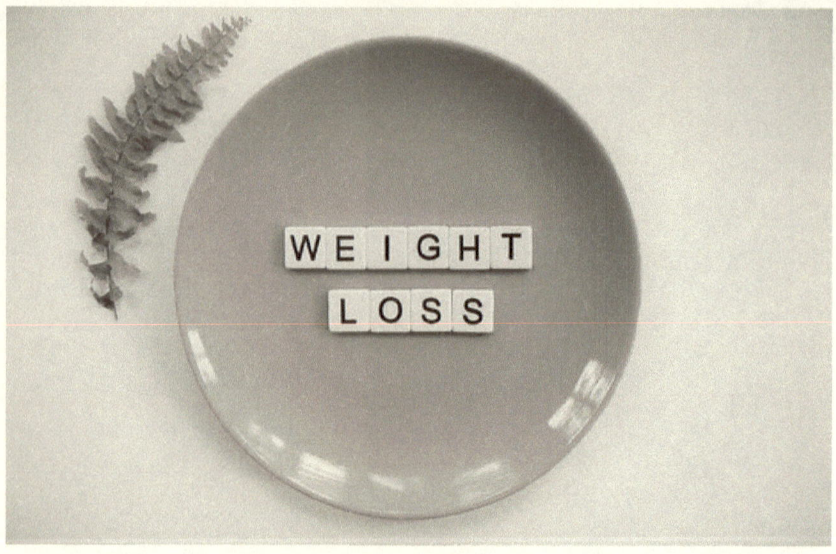

https://pixabay.com/photos/burn-fat-fat-burner-weight-loss-4235818/

As we talked about in chapter one, when you are on a ketogenic diet you place your body into a state known as Ketosis. This is caused when the liver produces ketones which permits fat to be burned into an energy source. The burning of fat is one of several advantages to the state of ketosis. Ketosis advances your complete state of health, making it a very successful instrument to aid you in losing weight.

People who do the Keto diet comment that they feel so much better while following this diet plan. They admit to having more energy as well as having higher mental and physical well-being. Being on a Keto diet plan also results in:

- Having less cravings for in-between meal snacks
- An overall decrease in the amount of calories consumed daily

- Having an increase in their self-control
- Greater energy levels which result in being more physically active

Even though these advantages to the Keto diet can result in weight loss, the Keto diet alone does not equal weight loss. In order for the Keto diet to be effective, one must keep precise, meticulous records of what their fat, protein, and carbohydrates daily consumption is. There needs to be equal amounts of the right macronutrients (protein, fat, and carbohydrates), weight loss goals that are realistic, as well as an accurate nutritional tracking system, in order to meet the goals you have set for your weight loss.

The Keto diet works to help you lose weight when your body reaches the Ketosis state. The way you do this is to eliminate carbohydrates and sugar from your diet.

The way the Keto diet supports and upholds ketosis is the secret to how the Keto diet work. You may be asking, "what is ketosis?" Ketosis is the state in which your body begins to use fat instead of glucose as its primary source for energy.

When you are trying to attain the state of Ketosis, which is the metabolic state that reduces the glucose your body stores within, also known as glycogen, which also lowers the levels of your blood sugar and insulin. Your body begins to seek another form of fuel to burn for energy uses.

How does the Keto diet compared against other diets like the Atkins diet, Mediterranean diet, and Paleo diet? There are similarities between the Keto diet and these other diets that we will now go over. The Keto diet has often been referred to as "the Atkins diet on steroids". The Atkins diet was originally called "The Atkins Nutritional Approach" which was created by Dr. Robert Atkins, a cardiologist. Intended to be an instrument for aiding in weight loss founded on the plan of "eating right, not less."

Keto Diet v The Atkins Diet

The Atkins Diet was created by Dr. Robert Atkins, was once called the "Atkins Nutritional Approach" was based on the idea that one should "eat right and not less." Some of the things that are like the keto diet is that one should cut down on the number of calories and carbohydrates you eat to get you to start eating healthier foods.

 The Keto and Atkins diet are similar because both diets lower carbohydrate and sugar intake and encourage the dieter to start eating foods that are whole and healthy. If these diets are done properly, the outcome is getting into the ketosis state and losing the weight you want, as well as gaining an improved mental sharpness along with a renewed physical vigor that comes from an increase in ketone fuel. The differences between the keto and Atkins diet is that the Atkins diet has four stages. The stages that most resemble the Keto diet are the first two--which are the orientation and harmonizing stages. The four stages of the Atkins diet are as follows:

- Stage 1: During the orientation stage you will set a goal to ingest a very low amount of carbohydrates, 20 to 25 of net carbohydrates is a good daily amount. You can gradually increase carbohydrate intake consumption until you are able to discover what the ideal amount of carbohydrates you can consume and avoid gaining weight.
- Stage 2: This is the stage in which you will want to create a sense of balance and maintaining a daily carbohydrate intake of 25 - 30 grams.
- Stage 3: This is the stage in which you will perfect the amount of net carbohydrates you can consume daily to get the results you are seeking. Usually the perfect daily carbohydrate amount is between 50 and 80 grams.
- Stage 4: When you get to this stage, you will be ready to maintain the daily carbohydrate numbers to maintain your net carbohydrates at 80 to 100 grams.

The Keto Diet v Paleo Diet

The Paleo or Paleolithic diet is also called the "caveman," "hunter-gatherer," or the
"Stone Age" diet. This diet is based on the consumption of the agricultural food from the prehistoric days of 10,000 years ago when our ancestors would gather and hunt.

No processed foods are allowed on the Paleo diet! Because milling wheat was not yet discovered, there is no food that is flour-based or sugars permitted.

This diet only allows foods that you hunt, catch, dig up, or pick from a tree or bush. Foods such as seafood, nuts, meat, vegetables, and fruits are what you may eat on a Paleo diet.

The way the Paleo diet is similar to the keto diet is that both diets forbid any starchy foods and recommend lots of vegetables that are non-starchy. Also, both diets place limits on the amounts of sugars, legumes, and grain you ingest as well as suggesting lots of animal proteins and fats that are of extreme quality.

Chapter 4
"Can a Ketogenic life reverse Diabetes and Prediabetes?"

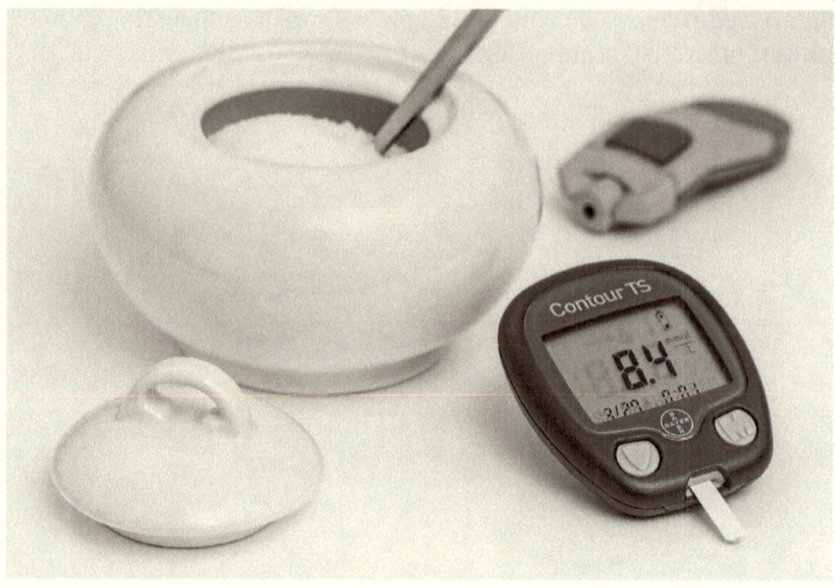

The answer to this question is "yes". Being on a ketogenic diet can help to lessen the symptoms of diabetes. Being on a high fat, low carbohydrate diet is certain to alter the way the body saves and utilizes its energy.

When on a ketogenic diet your body is going to change the fat grams you consume into energy. The Keto diet was first

discovered in 1924 as a means of treating epilepsy in children who were severely affected by the disease. Later studies have proven the keto diet is also an excellent means of treating type 2 diabetes.

What is Diabetes?

As one of the most common metabolic diseases in the U.S., the statistics for diabetes is currently growing. Since 2015 there have been 30.3 million Americans who have been diagnosed with this disease; that is 9.4% of the entire U.S. population. These figures are not even taking into account the number of people who are prediabetic or have never been diagnosed.

By making certain lifestyle and dietary changes, a person can help to reverse the effects of diabetes and slow down the progression of pre-diabetes becoming the full blown type 2 version of the disease.

The way you can do this is by starting a high-fat, low carbohydrate diet such as the keto diet. This type of diet has the possibly to completely reverse Type 2 diabetes by getting your blood sugar back on track.

Diabetes is the result of chronic high blood sugar. Your body naturally breaks down the carbohydrates eaten and turns it into glucose. This glucose is sent through the bloodstream in which your body then converts it to energy.

Unless you are in a state of ketosis, your body uses glucose as its primary source of energy.

The pancreas creates a hormone called insulin which is used to move the glucose through your cells to be turned into energy. If your body is unable to produce adequate insulin then the glucose just remains in the bloodstream and can result in diabetes.

How a high-fat/low-carb diet works

Most people that have type 2 diabetes are overweight; therefore, when we talk about a high fat, ketogenic diet being helpful to them, at first it does not make sense. However, the main idea of a high fat diet is to get the body to start burning fat as its primary energy source instead of carbohydrates.

The following are the benefits of the Keto diet:

- increased loss of fat
- improved body configuration

- improvement in brain activity
- decrease in swelling

Living a ketogenic lifestyle can do much more than just help you lose the excess weight you have been fighting to lose for so long. It can also help you to think with more clarity, and can even aid people that have diabetes to not resist insulin and to get their blood sugar in order once and for all.

When on a high-fat/ low-carb ketogenic diet you should not eat a lot of saturated fats. This means that you should ensure the fat you ARE eating is "heart-healthy". The following foods are considered to be healthy "fats":

- eggs
- salmon and other similar fish
- cottage cheese
- avocado
- olives and olive oil
- nut butter
- certain nuts
- seeds

When you are on a ketogenic diet you have the possibility to lower glucose readings. If you have type 2 diabetes it is imperative that you watch the amount of carbohydrates you consume because carbohydrates turn to sugar, which can ultimately result in blood sugar levels spiking too high. When you change the dietary focus to fats instead of carbohydrates, you will eventually end up with a decreased level of blood sugar.

Chapter 5
"What are other benefits of the Keto Lifestyle?"

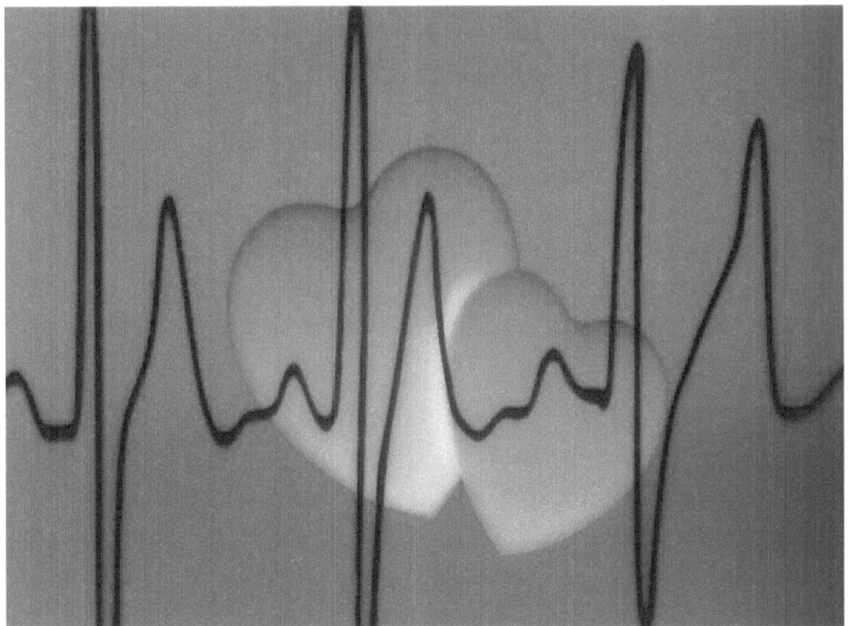

The keto diet is all the buzz on social media and people are bragging about the dramatic weight loss results they are recognizing from this diet. Besides weight loss, what are the other benefits of the Keto diet and lifestyle? The most important benefit of being on the keto diet is the amount of energy you will have, as well as an increased ability to overcome many physical ailments.

There are nine known benefits to the keto diet, such as:

- lowered case of inflammation
- improvement on the ability to burn fat grams
- a renewed sense of mental clarity and/or sharpness
- an unlimited supply of energy you didn't know you had

- complexion that is clearer
- decreased amount of cravings
- Mitochondrial biogenesis
- lowering your chance for chronic disease
- increase in anti-aging effects

The primary benefits you get from being on a ketogenic diet are the anti-inflammatory and mitochondrial stimulation benefits. What is mitochondrial biogenesis and it benefits and affects? A question you might now be asking yourself. It is the process the cells go through to create new mitochondria. This is how the cells learn to adapt to the ever changing environmental and physiological conditions.

Certain conditions, such as restricted caloric intake (when dieting) or an increase in energy requirements (when exercising) forces the body's cells to adjust their metabolic process which aids in preserving the energy levels available to the needs of the tissues and cells.

The ketogenic diet is therapeutic because the way the body is filled with the many nutrients that this diet offers.

Guaranteeing the foods you eat are fats from clean protein sources will benefit most on the Keto diet. Additionally, make certain vegetables and herbs you consume are rich in antioxidants. The blend of antioxidant vegetables and herbs, and healthy fats will be completely therapeutic to this new dietetic lifestyle.

Let us discuss the benefits of this new ketogenic lifestyle:

A ketogenic diet will literally turn your body into a machine that burns fat. The way this happens is by putting your body into a state known as "ketosis". This happens once the body starts burning fat (not carbs) as its energy source. Once you have been following the keto diet a few days, you will start burning the fat you eat as energy which puts your body in the ketosis state. Those new to the keto diet can learn if they are in ketosis by using a urine ketone strip or blood prick meter. Once you become more accustomed to the keto diet, you will be able to tell on your own by how your body responds whether you are in ketosis.

When you are on a low carbohydrate diet, you will feel less hungry. The reason for this is because this type of diet tends to automatically decrease the appetite. Research has proven that when carbohydrate numbers are reduced and the amount of protein and fat consumed is increased, the result is a lowered amount of total daily caloric intake.

People lose a lot more weight, more quickly, when they are on a low carbohydrate diet rather than when they are on a low-fat diet.

Chapter 6
"Foods that you should avoid in the Keto Lifestyle"

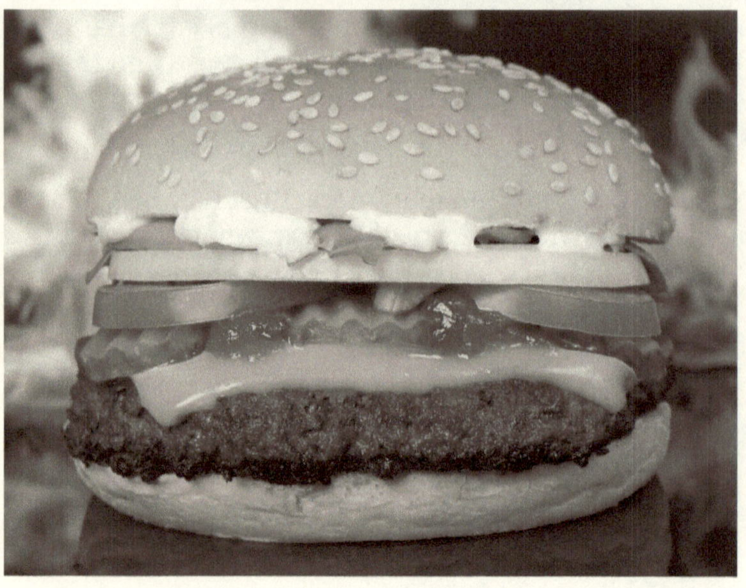

When you start a keto lifestyle, you must know there are several foods that should be absolutely avoided. The breakdown of foods you should eat when on a Keto diet include the following;

- 70-80 % fats
- 5-10 % carbohydrates
- 20-25 % proteins

Carbohydrates that are a "no-no" when on the keto diet include the following:

- Wheat, barley, rye, corn, barley, oats, rice, quinoa, millet, sorghum, bulgur, sprouted grains, and buckwheat.
- Also you must avoid any breads, cookies, pastas, crackers, and pizza crusts made from the above ingredients must all be avoided.

Additionally, keto dieters should avoid the following beans and legumes:

- Kidney beans, chickpeas, black beans, lentils, green peas, lima, pinto, white, cannaline, fava beans, and black-eye peas.

For the most part, the following fruits should only be eaten in moderation when on the keto diet:

- One small banana, ½ cup pineapple, 1 small papaya, 1 medium apple and orange, 1 cup of grapes, and a medium tangerine or mango.
- All fruit juices--except for one cup of orange juice
- Any dried fruits like dates, raisins, and dried mangos (can have a cup of raisins)
- Fruit juice concentrates- except for 2 fluid ounces of apple juice concentrate

Vegetables that contain a lot of starch should be strictly avoided! Starchy veggies are full of carbohydrates that turn to sugar and will make you gain weight. The following veggies contain starch:

- Yams, sweet potatoes, potatoes (but you may have one small baked potato, occasionally) carrots, peas, parsnips, yucca (except ½ cup of raw yucca), corn and cherry tomatoes (except for 1 cup of raw cherry tomatoes).

Any form of sugar or it derivatives are not allowed when on the keto diet. We are all aware what sugar does when it is consumed. The following items are considered to be sugars and are absolutely not allowed:

- Honey, agave nectar, raw sugar, maple syrup, turbinado sugar, high fructose corn syrup and cane sugar.

There are also some protein foods that can do damage to your keto lifestyle such as milk, low-fat dairy products and animal products that are factory-farmed.

Milk should be avoided--however, you can have some raw milk or a ½ cup of whole milk. Shredded cheese products--this often has potato starches contained within it. It is okay to have ½ cup of shredded cheese on occasion.

Fat-free or reduced fat dairy products are not allowed; this includes fat-free/substitution butter products. However, you can consume ½ cup of whole milk.

The following animal products that are factory farmed include:

- Meats that were grain fed, fish that has been farmed within a factory, hot dogs, salami, sausages that are packaged,beef jerky, corned beef, canned meats, smoked, cured, and salted meats. You must also avoid chicken nuggets, bacon, and fish sticks.

Even though the keto diet is all about high-fat intake, there are still certain fats that must never be consumed. This includes the following:

- Avoid the following oils at all costs: canola, soybean,corn, grapeseed, sesame, peanut, sunflower and safflower.

When on the keto diet, there are also certain beverages and drinks that must be avoided. This includes:

- Alcohol: beer (12 fluid ounces), wines- especially sweet wines, (you can have *one* glass of sweet dessert wine), cocktails, mixer drinks with fruit juices in them, syrups and sodas that are flavored, and flavored liquors.
- The following sweet/sugary beverages are also forbidden: all sodas that are sweetened with sugar and diet sodas-- the reason is that the sweeteners contained in diet sodas can interrupt the ketosis process, blood sugar,as well as boost cravings.
- Fruit and vegetable juices, also any bottled or fresh juices. Coffee or tea with sweet milk or sweeteners added to it.
- Any dairy or dairy replacement products; this also includes milk sweetened products.

In addition to the above listed products, one should avoid any packaged or processed foods when on a keto diet. This includes any cookies or cakes that have been baked commercially. Also, margarines, candies, and food with carrageenan in it. Avoid ice cream, wheat gluten, sodas, soft drinks, and especially FAST FOOD!!

There are 108 foods that will slow down or shut the process of your bodies ability to burn fat. In order to stay in ketosis, you must keep your total carb intake to a minimum of 20-30 grams of net carbs daily. Consuming too many carb-rich foods can take you out of ketosis and decrease your body's ability to burn fat.

Chapter 7
"What to do if you have the Keto Flu"

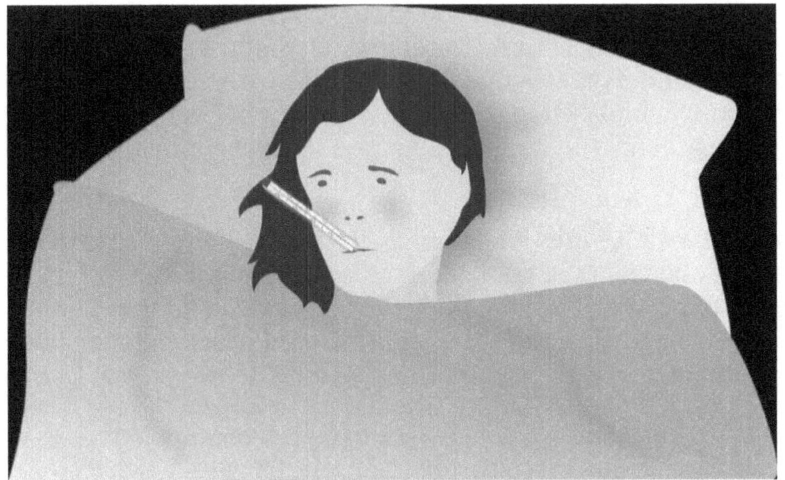

https://pixabay.com/vectors/influenza-flu-fever-grippe-cold-156098/

You know what the regular influenza is and what to do to get rid of it or even prevent it. However, have you ever heard of the ketogenic flu? What are the symptoms, causes and how to get rid of it? This next chapter is going to be all about what to do if you should have the keto flu. The keto flu has many of the same symptoms as the regular flu, and it is the result of your body going into the state of ketosis.

When you start the keto diet, the objective is to drastically reduce your carbohydrate intake and substitute it with fats and protein. The result of the changes in ones diet causes a metabolic state known as ketosis.

There are certain foods (mentioned in the previous chapter) that the keto dieters must avoid. These foods are anything that contain sugars--such as cakes, grains, and starches like rice and grains. No pasta, beans, fruits, or root vegetables (like carrots or potatoes) and absolutely no alcohol.

The Keto diet includes such foods such as chicken, turkey, beef, bacon, fish that is fatty such as salmon or trout. It also allows eggs, butter, healthy oils, avocados, and unprocessed cheeses.

Our bodies are trained to naturally burn carbohydrates for energy; however, when on the keto diet you stop consuming carbohydrates in order to start burning fat for energy. This is called ketosis. It is when the body stops burning carbohydrates and starts burning ketones for energy. Sometimes this switch is too much and it creates flu-like symptoms which is the bodies reaction to withdrawing from a lack of carbohydrates. The keto flu causes feelings of nausea, diarrhea, muscle cramps, and vomiting.

Symptoms of the keto flu generally begin just a few days into the diet; they last about a week, then go away--symptoms vary from person to person. The keto flu is the body's reaction to withdrawing from carbohydrate withdrawal which puts the body in a form of shock.

One experiences an adverse reaction to withdrawing from carbohydrates due to losing too many electrolytes which also causes dehydration. At least 25% of the people who go on the keto diet experience these keto-flu-like symptoms.

Symptoms vary from person to person. Some experiencing severe flu-like, to milder symptoms. Some of the more severe symptoms include headache, irritability, weakness, constipation, nausea, dizziness, vomiting, trouble sleeping, cramps, difficulty concentrating and sore muscles. All of these can begin just days after starting a new keto diet regimen.

As unpleasant as the keto flu is, there are ways to combat and heal that awful feeling so you will start feeling better quickly.

One of the main reasons you might get the keto flu is because of water. The carbohydrate known as Glycogen is stored in the water molecules of your body. Water is taken from your body very quickly when you start eliminating carbohydrates from your diet. You must remember to drink lots of water when you start the keto diet; otherwise you will become dehydrated--which causes

muscle cramps and fatigue--two of the symptoms suffered with
the keto flu.

Keto flu sufferers are low on electrolytes, the way to give these a
boost is to add some salt to your diet. Also, eat lots of green, leafy
vegetables, as well as avocados. Getting lots of sleep will give you
more energy which can also rid you of keto flu symptoms.

There are several things you can do to prevent the keto flu. The
best way is to transition your diet slowly; introducing more fats
(such as salmon and avocado) and removing the carbohydrates. If
you do this, your body is less likely to go into shock and develop
the keto flu.

Chapter 8
"How Do You Know if You Are in Ketosis?"

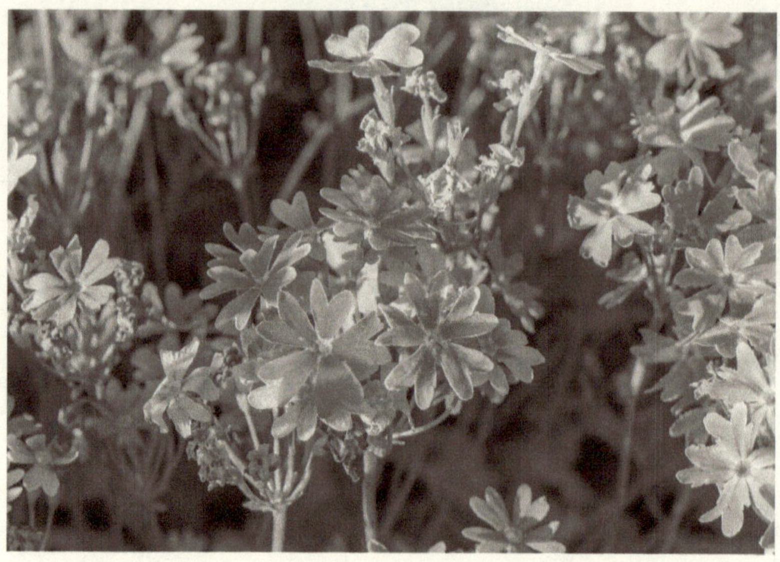

If you are looking for an effective way to lose weight, then you have come to the right place. The keto diet is the most popular way people everywhere are learning how to shed excess pounds in a fairly rapid manner.

The keto diet is an excellent way to advance your current state of health as well as lose weight. As long as you follow it accurately, this high fat, low carbohydrate diet plan will increase your levels of blood ketones. You will be amazed by this new source of fuel and the amount of energy you will have as well as the one of a kind health benefits you will get from the keto diet.

When you enter into the ketosis state, there are 10 signs and symptoms you have arrived (some of these are not positive). In the next section we have listed these symptoms:

1. **Bad Breath**: many people on the ketogenic or Atkins diet have reported that their breath has a fruity smell to it. The reason for this, is the elevated levels of ketones.

Often, people will combat this breath issue with sugar-free gum or sugar-free drinks. If you do this, you must check the carbohydrate count.

2. **Weight loss**: low carbohydrate dies, such as the keto diet offer efficient ways to lose weight. When doing the keto diet you will experience both long and short term weight loss. During the first week of the keto diet, you experience a lot of weight loss--many believe this to be fat loss, However, it is mostly water and stored carb loss.

3. **Increase of Ketones in your blood:** The main objective of the keto diet is to reduce the blood sugar and advance the ketones. As you progress along in this diet, you will begin burning those ketones and fat as the main source of energy your body uses. The best way to calculate ketones in your blood is with the use of a special meter. This meter will gauge the amount of Beta-hydroxybutyrate (BHB) that is showing in your blood. BHB are the main ketones that appear in your blood when in ketosis. Keto experts comment that the ideal amount of BHB levels should be from 0.5 - 3.0 mmol/L. Gauging one's blood for ketones is the best way to get an accurate account for the number of ketones in the blood. The negative side, you must prick your finger to access the blood sample.

4. **Advanced amount of ketones appear in you breath or urine:** You can also gauge the number of ketones in your blood with the use of a breathalizer. This tool actually gauges the acetone in your breath; when your body is in a ketosis state, acetone is one of the three main elements present. An acetone breath analyzer is very efficient; however, it is always a better reading when blood is gauged. Lastly, if you are looking for an inexpensive, quick method to gauge the ketones in your body, there is also the urine method.

5. **Suppresses the appetite:** A lowered appetite is often what people on the keto diet report. The reason for this is still under current study; most of these studies find that the increase in ketones decreases one's appetite.

6. **Your energy and focus is increased:** When first starting out on the keto diet it has been reported by dieters they feel "brain fog", increased fatigue, as well as ill. However, long term keto dieters who have turned keto into their new lifestyle report an unbelievable advancement in their energy levels and mental focus. When starting on a low-carb regimen, your body must learn how to burn fat instead of carbs for energy. When you are in ketosis, your brain begins burning ketones rather than glucose as its energy source. Ketones are an intoxicating source of energy for our brain. Ketones have even been experimented medically for treating brain disorders such as concussions and loss of memory. It's no wonder why people who have been on the keto diet for long term use experience a sharper memory with better clarity and brain performance.

7. **Temporary Weariness:** A temporary weariness is one of the biggest complaints people have when they first start the keto journey. These fatigued feeling is often the reason many people quit the diet before they have had a chance to fully experience its benefits. These side effects are completely normal; you must remember that your body has been accustomed to using carbs for energy, therefore, it will take some adjusting to get used to no carbs. It can take anywhere from a week to an entire month for ketosis to take place. You can cut down on the fatigue you feel by taking electrolyte supplements until you have reached full ketosis. When you cease the consumption of processed foods you are also eliminating a lot of salt from your diet. Since salt retains water, you are also going to lose water; hence, electrolytes. You should try adding the following supplements to your diet: 2,000-4,000 mg. of sodium; 1000 mg of potassium; and 300 mg of magnesium daily.

8. **Temporary decrease in performance:** The removal of carbohydrates from our diet initially causes a lowered performance rate in exercising at first. However, this is only a temporary problem; after a few weeks it slowly begins to return. The reason for the decreased performance is because the muscle's glycogen store levels have been lowered; the is the primary energy source the muscle's use when doing intense exercise routines. After a few weeks on the keto diet, it was reported that people

had an overwhelming increase in their overall endurance during strenuous exercise.

9. **Issues with digesting food:** When you begin the keto diet your are creating some changes in your diet which also affects your digestive tract. Some of the biggest issues with digestion can be constipation and diarrhea. Once your body has adjusted to the diet, these digestive issues should subside. However, it would be a good idea to keep a list of the types of food that brings on these issues to prevent future flair ups. Another way to prevent digestive issues from occurring is to consume plenty of low carb, healthy vegetables. Also, ensure to keep diversity in your diet--by doing so, you lower the chance of digestive issues and nutritional deficiencies.

10. **Inability to sleep:** People who first start the keto diet find it difficult to get a good night's sleep. New keto dieter's complain they wake up in the middle of the night craving carbs when they first start eliminating them from their diet. However, people who have reached ketosis are amazed at how good they sleep at night.

Chapter 9
"Keto Diet and Macros"

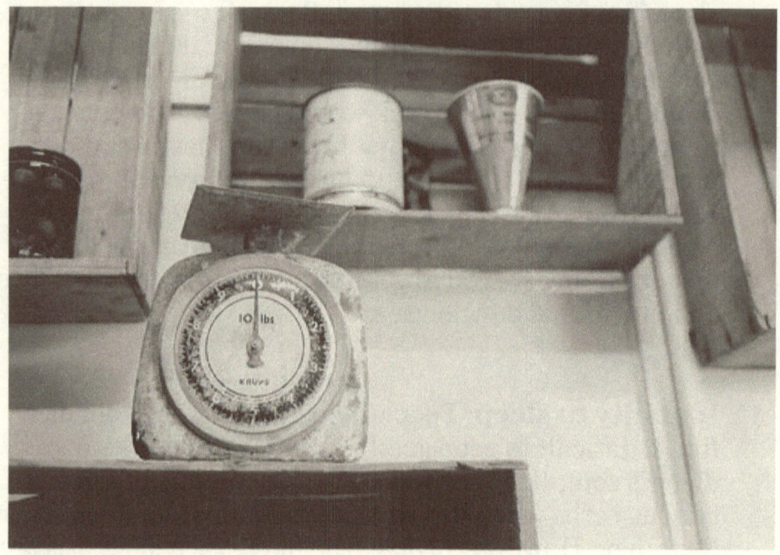

Anyone who wants to start the keto diet needs to know about counting macros. When we speak about counting macros, we mean the counting of daily carbs, fat, and protein grams. This can be a lot more difficult than one might think at first. Your whole keto diet plan depends on your counting macros correctly.

You need to ensure not too many carbs and just the right amount of fat--if either of these numbers are incorrect you will not reach ketosis--and lose less weight. This section is going to cover how to count and keep track of your macros while on the keto diet to ensure you the most efficient weight loss.

When counting your daily macros you need to keep in mind that you stick to the following: 60-75 % fat grams; 5-10 % carbohydrates; and 15-30 % protein grams. Now that you know the percentages of each that needs to be in your daily diet; how do you figure the number of daily grams of each? Well, let's take a 1600 daily diet plan as an example.

You need to know the following information in converting calories to grams:

- Carbohydrates have 4 grams per calorie
- There are nine calories per each fat gram
- Four calories per each gram of protein

If you are shooting for the standard keto diet plan--10% carbohydrates, 20% protein, and 70% fat. You can follow the equations below to determine the number of grams you need of each in order to successfully reach ketosis.

- Daily carb intake: Take 1600 (daily caloric intake) x .10 (10%) divided by 4 (number of grams per calorie) = 40 grams of carbs each day
- Daily fat intake would be figured as: 1600 x .70 (70%) divided by 9 = 125 fat grams per day
- Daily protein is determined by: 1600 x .20 (20%) divided by 4 = 80 protein grams per day.

Of course, it is most imperative to keep precise track of your daily carb intake. Tracking protein and fat is a bit more accommodating to your preference. For instance, when determining the adequate amount of daily protein, you should take your ideal weight-- say 150 pounds and divide in half--75 grams would be your ideal daily protein grams intake. The remainder of your daily intake should be fat grams; eat enough fat grams to make you feel full. That can be as much as 125 grams of fat, if necessary.

For those of you who find math a bit of a challenge, you can always tally your daily macros using an app on your mobile device called a "cron-o-meter". Just remember, whichever method you choose for tracking macros needs to be the one you consistently stick with. You need to show a commitment to the keto diet and the best way to do so is committing to tracking macros efficiently.

Now that you have a basic idea about how to track your macros you are almost ready to begin your new journey and lifestyle. Once you get the hang of the keto lifestyle, and you begin to feel the benefits of eating this way, you will wonder what took you so long?

Chapter 10
"The Dangers of the Keto Diet"

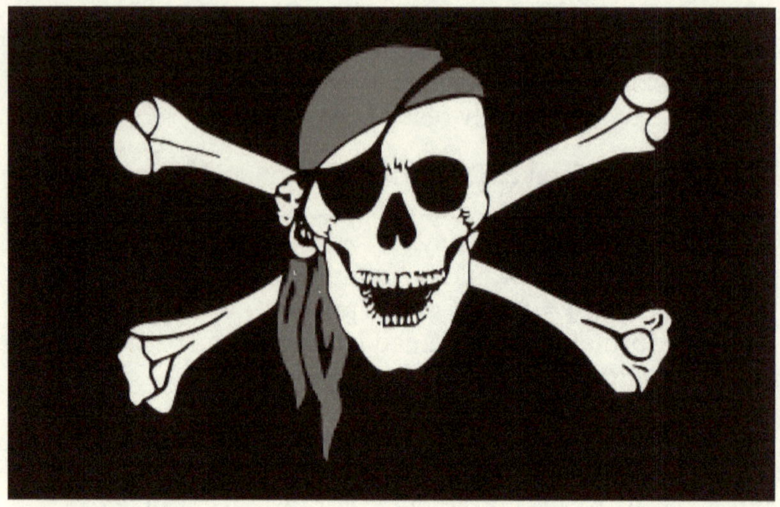

https://pixabay.com/vectors/pirate-crossbones-skull-flag-bones-47705/

The Keto diet has become one of the most popular ways to lose weight. High-fat, low carb eating plan; however, doctors are still having their doubts about whether this is a safe diet plan. Coming up next we are going to go over some of the known dangers to the keto diet.

You may think the ketogenic diet is a new diet fad; however, in reality it has actually been around since the 1920s. Originally used as a way to treat patients with epilepsy, it is now boasted has being a treatment for anything from infertility to type II diabetes.

Dieticians and doctors both admit that Keto is an excellent way to drop those excess pounds; people are losing up to 10 pounds in a short time of only a few weeks. However, most early weight loss is mainly water and not real fat.

The way the ketogenic diet works by cutting daily carb intake to less than 50 carbs per day. Replacing those carbs with fat and protein, this puts the body in a state known as ketosis in which you burn fat for an energy source.

Many of the people who do the Keto diet like it because it is strict without all the guesswork of the typical diet plan. However, as easy as it seems to comply with a keto diet, it appears only about 45% of its participants actually are able to follow it completely. The reason for such a low percentage is mainly because people do not want to deal with the side effects, the feeling of being isolated from society because they cannot eat what others are eating, and the biggest thing--cravings for food with carbs.

Below are 11 of the top concerns doctors and dieticians have regarding the keto diet that everyone should be aware of before they start a keto regimen.

1. There can be considerable muscle loss as one of the side effects of the keto diet. Ongoing research has found that even though keto dieters continuously workout and do resistance training, they are still losing muscle mass. The reason is not yet known; but one belief is that protein alone does not build muscle in the same way as protein and carbs do. Following a study done in March 2018 *Sports* journal, people lost the same amount of body fat and increase muscle as those on other diets did. But there was one difference, the people on the keto diet DID LOSE more leg muscle mass than the other group did.

Chapter 11
"Exercise and the Keto Diet"

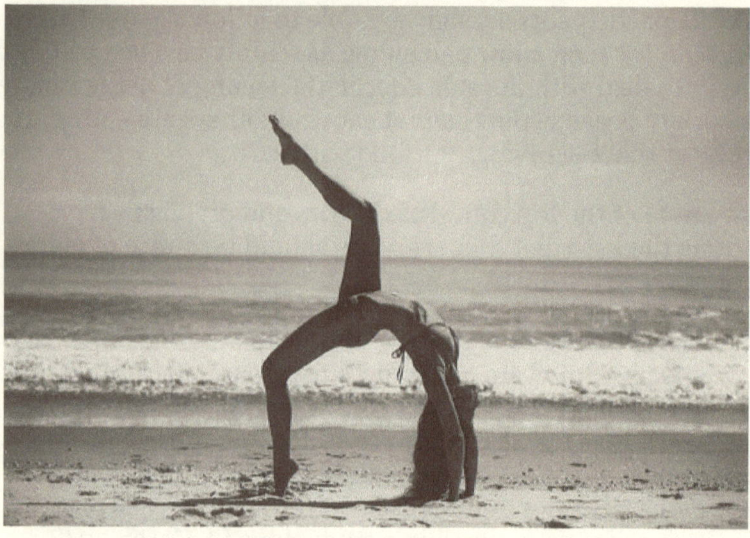

As you are aware exercising works best at boosting your weight loss as well as maintaining high levels of energy. You know that you must cut the carb intake in order to get in a ketosis state. As well, since carbohydrates are no longer the principal source of energy, you need to learn what options there are for exercising when in a state of ketosis.

Exercise while dieting is good for your health. It is good for your heart, creates lean, toned muscles, as well as strengthening the bones. When in ketosis there is a way to effectively create an exercise regimen with just a few considerations to keep in mind.

Exercising while in Ketosis

There is some good news to the keto dieters regarding exercising. Exercise is a total possibility. There are also many energetic and healthy benefits to exercising when on a keto diet.

When setting up an exercise plan while in Ketosis you need to ensure you are eating enough to give you sufficient energy.

Low intensity cardio exercise is what most health care experts recommend a person on the keto diet to take part in. Some examples of low intensity exercise is jogging, swimming, cycling and recreational sports. Weight lifting. by using lighter weights and fewer reps is also a good exercise for a keto dieters.

Type of Exercise

Depending on your nutritional requirements, your exercise regimen is going to vary. There are four basic styles of exercises: aerobic, anaerobic, stability, and flexibility.

- The aerobic exercise- is about low intensity, long duration, and the burning of fat
- Anaerobic exercise- is short duration, weight lifting/HIIT, and intensely high fat burning exercises
- Flexibility exercises- this is yoga, support, stretching, soft-tissue, and an advancement of range of motion exercises
- Stability exercises- these are exercises that focus on core training and balance; supporting alignment, body control, and increased balance

Getting started with an exercise regimen when on the keto diet:

When you first begin the keto diet you might not feel like exercising. The primary reason for this is the "keto flu" making its way through your body during the first week or two of the diet. Exercises that require high intensity--like weight-lifting, sprinting, or HIIT--are going to be more strenuous. The reason is that the fat you have been using for energy/fuel is not as easily accessible as the carbs once were to your muscles.

In addition, these high intensity workouts are going to cause you to tire out much quicker than before. As well, you will not have the endurance you once had, causing you to "hit a wall" early into the workout.

The answer to this is low-intensity aerobic exercise. Some low-intensity workouts include--yoga, bike riding, and jogging. During the first couple weeks of the keto diet engaging in low-intensity workouts will help get your body in shape as it gets accustomed to burning fat for fuel instead of carbs.

Once your body is used to the keto regimen, you can eventually work your way back up to those high intensity workouts. Just do not over-do it.

Chapter 12
"Frequently Asked Questions"

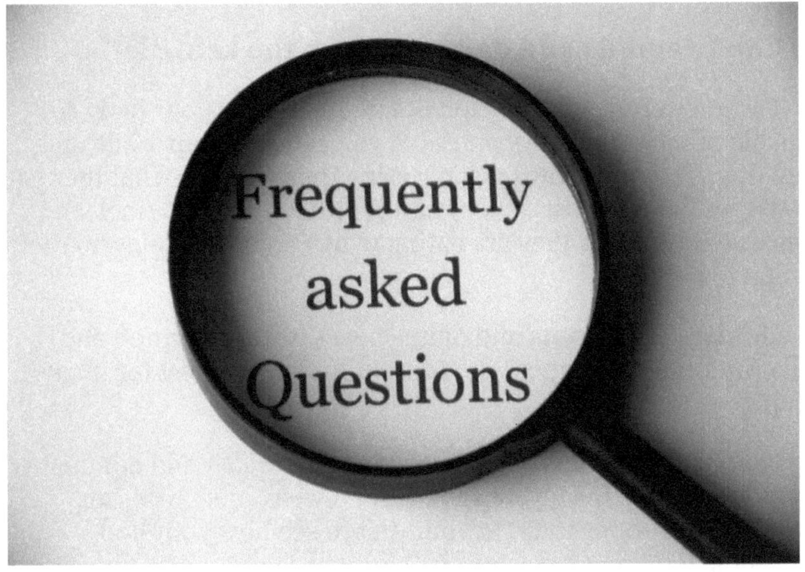

https://www.pexels.com/photo/black-and-white-business-career-close-up-221164/

Q: What is the Ketogenic (Keto) diet?

A: A ketogenic diet is a diet plan that involves a very low intake of carbohydrates. Typically a person following this regimen consumes no more than 30 grams of carbohydrates. As a result, when on a Ketogenic diet you will be ingesting lots of fats that are heart-healthy along with a small amount of healthy protein sources.

If bacon, eggs, avocado, cheese, and steak are some of your favorite foods then you are going to do well on the Keto diet.

Q: When on a Ketogenic diet, what is it doing to your body?

A: When we talk about a "Ketosis state" we are referring to how your body (mainly the liver) digests the ketones in your body. Ketones are organic substances in your body that when they are processed by your body they put your body in this state of ketosis.

When the amount of carbohydrates you ingest are decreased, your body is going to require another energy source. When on the Keto diet, your body begins to utilize fats at a source of fuel because there is very little glucose available.

Q: Can I eat nuts and dairy when on the keto diet?

A: The answer to this question is Yes. As long as your body is capable of handling dairy and nuts you can eat them while on a keto diet. The only drawback to eating these foods is that they can be trigger foods--most dieters find it difficult to keep track and measure how much they are eating which creates a delay in their weight loss.

In addition, eating nuts and dairy causes water retention and inflammation. Also, these foods are difficult to digest for many people.

If your weight loss has been delayed at all; you should eliminate these food items from your diet. After a week or so, you can slowly re-introduce them to your diet to see how your body responds.

Q: Is it OK to drink alcohol while on the Keto diet?

A: Yes. It is not a good idea to drink alcohol that has high-carbs-- such as beer, sweet wine, and cocktails--however, it is fine to partake in a glass or two of dry wine or pure liquor.

Many keto dieters have recognized their tolerance to alcohol is much lower; so, if you are going to drink any alcohol, ensure that you take it easy at first.

Additionally, keep in mind there a calories in alcohol, so if your goal on keto is losing weight ensure you track these calories.

Q: Is it necessary to track calories and macros when on the keto diet?

A: When you first start the keto diet it is important to track calories and macros--at least until you get accustomed to it. Carbs are tricky and can sneak up on you from nowhere.

The way you can ensure you do not go over your daily allotment of carbs is to track and measure EVERYTHING!

The way you can do this is to purchase a food scale and an app that is for tracking--this way you can ensure you are eating the right amounts and staying on track.

When counting calories for weight loss you need to create a calorie deficit. The way you do this is to come up with a daily number of calories you need for maintenance--then subtract 15% - 20% until you reach the caloric goal. When you set a larger deficit, you will lose weight more quickly; however, it will be more difficult to maintain this deficit. On the other hand, a lower deficit results in slower weight loss, but it is less stress on your mind and body.

Q: How much protein is allowable?

A: The preservation of muscle mass is very important when dieting; therefore, you need to ensure you consume plenty of protein. The precise amount of protein you should be eating is dependent on your current muscle mass, level of activity, as well as your personal goals and preferences.

The general rule for protein consumption should be from 0.68 to 1 gram for each pound of lean body mass. The way you determine lean body mass is your body weight minus fat.

Q: What is a good amount of fat to consume?

A: The amount of fat you consume should be considered a leverage on the amount of your daily caloric intake. Putting it in easier terms, the amount of fat you consume is going to replace the amount of carbs you once consumed.

If your goal on the keto diet is to lose weight then you will not need to consume copious fat amounts; these fat sources should come from what is stored in your body.

For example, if you are on a 1600 calorie diet, you need to consume 25 net grams of carbs and 117 grams of protein.

There are 4 calories in each gram of carbs and protein, and a gram of fat has 9 calories. Therefore, you will be consuming the following: (25 / 117) x 4 = 142 x4 =568 calories from carbs and protein and 1092 calories from fat, (114 grams).

It is ok not to meet the fat macro as long as you are not hungry; however, it is imperative for you to meet your protein macro.

Q: Is the Keto diet an effective way to lose weight? If so, what makes it effective?

A: The answer is YES. The Keto diet has been proved to be one of the most effective plans for losing weight. The reason for this is that with the keto diet your are creating a lower caloric deficit without excessive hunger; while permitting greater accessibility to stored fat.

In addition, people who have done the keto diet claim they have a lot more energy which allows for them to move around and be more active throughout the day.

Q: Is the Keto diet the same thing as a low-carb diet?

A: The keto diet is a form of low-carb diet. When we speak of a diet being low-carb it means the diet restricts carbohydrates. The keto diet is a little more restrictive in that net carbs are limited to 20-25 per day (the stricter version) or 100-120 carbs per day.

Q: Isn't a lot of fat in the diet unhealthy?

A: Surprisingly, the answer to this question is no. Fat is not something you should be afraid of consuming. Additionally, saturated fats do have a healthy place in heart health.

The fat you should avoid, however, is *processed* fats. This is soybean and canola oils as well as *trans fat*.

Fats derived from meat and eggs, as well as fats such as avocado, coconut, and olive oil are healthy fats and you should not be afraid of consuming these fats.

Chapter 13
"How to Save Money on the Keto Diet"

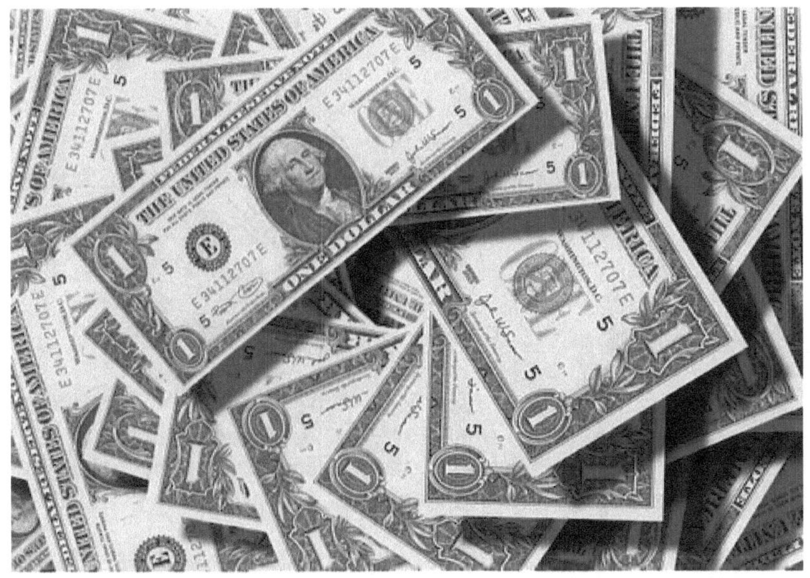

https://pixabay.com/photos/dollar-currency-money-us-dollar-499481/

So you are ready to start the keto diet? However, your biggest fear now is that it is going to cost a lot of money to buy low-carb foods. We all know that the cheapest foods are loaded with carbohydrates.

This is a true statement to a point. However, there are ways to get by this. Following a ketogenic diet regimen does not have to be an expensive endeavor. There are a few strategies you can use to lower the cost of being on a keto diet to fit your budget.

Below are some ways to save money on the keto diet:

- Clip coupons
- Look for deals on your keto foods
- Purchase items in bulk

- Make extra food and freeze it for later
- Shop ahead of time by planning for the week's meals
- Buy frozen fruits & vegetables
- Shop for seasonal foods
- Buy a membership at a wholesale club store (Costco, Sam's Club)

Tips to implement on how to save money on Keto:

1. **You should buy all your keto supplies in bulk**

   Buying food and other supplies in bulk is always the best way to save money. It can be easier to shop at the local grocery store; however, you will not save as much at the grocery store as at Costco, WalMart, or Sam's Club.

   Another affordable store is Aldi and Trader Joe's (owned by the same owner). Also, seek out farmer's markets for farmers or butchers who offer CSA / prescription-based programs for shopping.

   Whenever you discover something on sale or offered at a good price by it in bulk. Buy all your seasonings, coconut milk, and other essential items for the pantry in bulk--this will save money over buying it a la carte.

   When you find meat on sale, buy it in quantity and freeze for later. Buy frozen vegetables instead of fresh produce. You can purchase several bags of frozen vegetables and make a quick stir-fry m, such

   In addition, you should by all your fats in bulk form, such as:

   - Organic extra virgin coconut oil
   - Extra virgin olive oil
   - Avocado oil
   - Grass-fed butter
   - Ghee

With a 2-year shelf life for coconut oil, you can save a lot of money by purchasing it in bulk when it is on sale. This is a lot smarter than buying smaller portions whenever you need it. Also, you buy coconut oil try to find product that is in glass containers; if you cannot find it in a glass container you can transfer it to a mason jar. Glass containers ensures the fat is not absorbed by the plastic container--even it is is BPA-free plastic. Additionally, when you store fat products in a cool, dark place it preserves the life of the product, keeping it from going bad.

Chapter 14
"Advice or Takeaways"

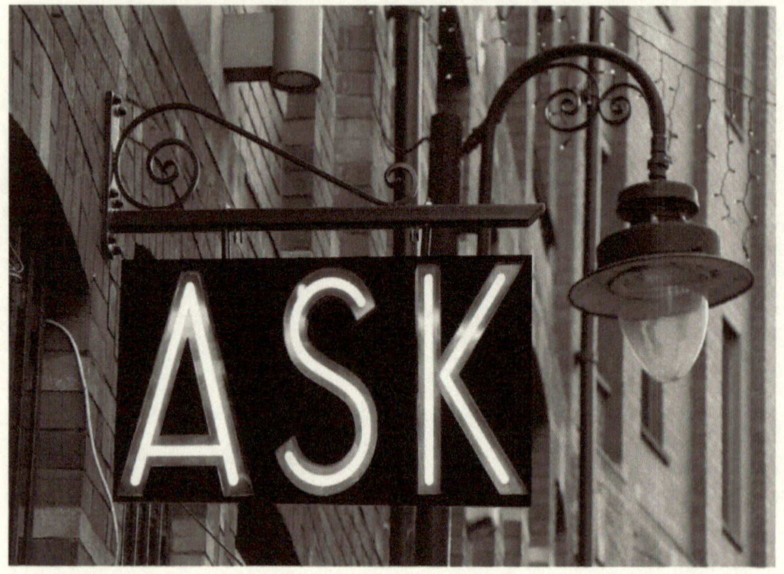

https://pixabay.com/photos/ask-sign-design-creative-2341784/

The final chapter of this keto book is going to discuss what the keto diet plan is about. This is diet plan involves a regimen that is all about a mediocre amount of fats and protein, combined with very little carbohydrates.

When starting a ketogenic diet, you are about to begin a life that is a continuous process. This process is one in which your body adapts to a living on a high fat consumption diet.

As you have read in the previous pages it is not about being on a diet. This plan is a change in lifestyle. The Keto diet is a plan to help you learn how to live healthy, eating healthier is how to start.

This next chapter is intended to give you 10 of the most imperative tips for being successful when on the Keto diet. These tips are meant to aid you and clarify any former misconceptions and give you a real plan of attack for losing weight and keeping it off.

1. **The first tip is to know what to keep your main focus on.**

    Should it be calories, carbs, or fat and protein grams? The way you can be the most successful when dieting is to find a diet that is very little calories yet it reduces cravings and hunger. Only then will you be able to lose weight successfully.

2. **Only eat foods and use ingredients that are Keto.**

    This means keeping your carb intake below 35 grams; and net carbs under 25 grams. Try to keep it lower than 20 grams of carbs if you want to seek the true benefits of achieving ketosis and losing the maximum amount of weight.

Below is a list of foods you should and should not eat:

Foods you *should* eat include:

- Meats such as: fish, eggs, lamb, beef, poultry, etc.
- Vegetables that are low in carbs--such as: broccoli, spinach, kale, cauliflower,
- Dairy with high fat content--hard cheese, hard fat cream, butter..
- Nuts & seeds- macadamia, sunflower, walnuts, ets.
- Avocados & berries--raspberries, blackberries, and any other impact berries that are low-glycemic
- Sweeteners such as erythritol, stevia, monk fruit, as well as any other sweeteners that are low in carbs
- Fats such as coconut oils, high fat salad dressing, saturated fats

Foods that you *should not* eat include:

- Tubers--this is potatoes, yams, and anything similar
- Fruit--bananas, apples, oranges, etc.
- Sugar--honey, maple syrup, & agave, etc.
- Grains--rice, wheat, and corn

3. **Make sure you keep accurate track of your Macros:**

    You need to make sure you are accurately tracking your daily caloric intake. You can do this by using an app that tracks calories as well as a good scale. When you use both of these tools, you will ensure an accurate account of what you are eating and therefore, better weight loss results.

Certain things to look for in a good scale:

- Make sure there is a button for **_converting weights_**-- such as grams/ounces, etc.
- **_Automatic shut-off_** --if the scale you purchase for measuring food has an automatic shut-off, this can create issues. Make sure this feature has a manual or programmable shut- off feature to the automatic shut-off.
- **_Tare function-_** when a scale allows one to have the capability of weighing the utensil, bowl or plate the food is on first it becomes much more useful of an item.
- **_Features a plate that is removable_**--this is an invaluable feature; particularly for cleaning messy foods you might weigh

Now that you have a scale for accurate weighing, you will find it is much easier to lose weight.

However, do not forget that cheating on a diet is very simple if we don't watch our environment. Be extra careful and mindful when traveling--avoid restaurants that feature favorite foods that are excluded from your diet. Additionally, avoid buying "cheat" items at home--even if they are for other household members. Even though you have a strong will power, everyone has a weakness for something. Or, a day considered to be a "bad day" which is the perfect excuse to eat these foods.

Which brings us to #4 on this list of tips.

4. **Creating a different food environment**

    The Human race was not meant to sustain on the current food environment we live in. Eating unhealthy foods is way too easy.

    The every increasing bombardment of processed foods-- as well as a rapid decline in two-parent families--makes it easier to buy ready made foods that can quickly be heated in the microwave by a hungry teenager.

Ads for food, and yummy odors of restaurant food makes the part of our brain that was once used to hunt food lie dormant. It is now so much easier to get the foods we crave by picking up the phone and making a call to have it brought to us!

The way you keep this from occurring is to only have keto-friendly foods available in your home. Also, delete all restaurant phone numbers from your list of phone contacts in your cell. By removing these temptations, you will be less likely to cheat on your diet.

Plan you meals ahead of time. Prepare the weeks meals and freeze them in serving size containers. This way you can easily take one out and pop in the microwave when you are hungry. (Just as easily as you would a process meal).

Stay away from foods considered to be "convenient foods." If you like eating something and can binge on it, only have a small serving available to satisfy your craving.

Make it a rule that you can only eat what is tracked.

The use of these four tactics will ensure you new keto lifestyle is easy to follow. Eventually, you body and brain will seek out healthy alternatives to unhealthy eating. Therefore, resulting in more successful weight loss.

5. Seek advice of other Keto Dieters

Seeking the support of family and friends (new friends,too) that are also living a ketogenic lifestyle is one of the most overlooked tips to successful dieting. When you share your struggles, questions, and overcoming hurdles and triumphs with others you will see that you aren't the only one with these issues.

Listening to the success stories of other keto dieters will give you the inspiration needed to keep on and stay with this diet. Go online and seek out success stories other keto dieters have shared. Hearing the trials and tribulations of these people will give you the much needed encouragement you need to keep on going.

6. **Be alert for signs of the keto flu or other keto-related issues**

   Something to expect when suddenly limiting your carb intake are some unpleasant body changes at first. Because you are limiting your sodium intake you can expect to lose water weight first. This loss of water is going to create some flu-like symptoms. Such as:
   - cravings for sugar, sweets
   - dizziness
   - brain fog
   - unable to focus or concentrate
   - irritibility
   - stomach pain
   - nausea
   - cramping
   - confusion
   - sore muscles
   - insomnia

Many of these symptoms will vanish with the consumption of water or food that is filled with minerals. The idea here is to replenish the body with the lost water and minerals.

7. **The majority of keto foods should be homemade**
   You now are familiar with the why of the keto diet, and what you should eat as well as what to expect when on a keto diet. This step is going to help you to understand what precisely you should be eating.

   You can literally find hundreds of recipes for making breakfast, lunch, dinner, even deserts keto style. You can also find the infamous "fat bomb" recipes to satisfy those cravings for fat grams.

8. **Budget and plan each week ahead.**
   One of the most common myths regarding the keto diet is that it is expensive. However, in reality a days meals on this plan never goes over $8--(this is all inclusive of breakfast, lunch, dinner, dessert, and snacks)

Shopping for the meals on a keto diet is similar to shopping for other groceries:

- coupon clipping
- seeking out the deals
- schedule meals based on the deals of the week
- make recipes that have a lot of leftovers
- freeze meat and buy in bulk to freeze for later
- avoid buying impulse items

*There are more tips in the chapter about saving money.

9. **Do not alter your weight loss goals too rapidly.** The first week on the keto diet is going to net a lot of water weight loss. Additionally, your daily calories needs can alter with each passing day. One week you could lose 3-4 pounds, then go a few weeks with no loss at all. However, you must be patient and remain on the course of the diet.

As long as your average weight loss is 1-2 pounds a week you are on track for success. However, if you hit a weight loss plateau that lasts over a month, it is time to make some adjustments to the diet.

Here are some of the best strategies people on the Keto diet follow:

- Use the right calorie deficit (the higher the better if you have more body fat) when counting your macros
- Each month you should re-calculate your macronutrient needs --follow these new amounts
- Every two weeks you need to take a break from calorie deficits.
- Track keto foods by diligently remaining consistent-- ensure you don't cheat by tracking macros
- Try an intermittent fast
- Plan a fat fasting

If, after trying these strategies and you still don't beat the plateau--you may need to get checked for food allergies or sensitivities.

Finally, last but certainly not least is #10---

10. **Find a meal plan that works best for you and stick with it.**

Below are a few sample meal plans you can try--even though there are many plans you can find online:

Chapter 15
"Meal Plan for a Keto Diet"

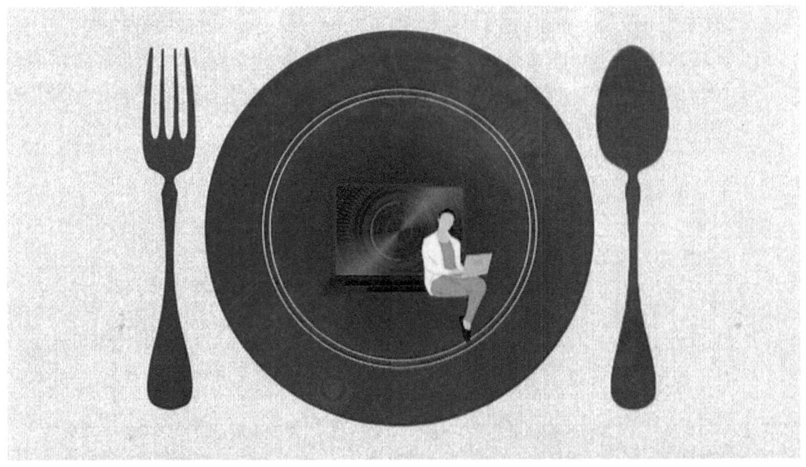

It is always a good idea to do meal prep whenever you are on a diet plan. The reason for this is that efficient meal preparation ensures you will be eating a diet that is balanced nutritionally. Efficient meal prep decreases any stress of what you should eat as well as ensuring you do not make any last minute, hurried decisions about what you are going to eat.

This next chapter provides you an entire week of meals for your new Keto diet. Each day has breakfast, lunch, dinner, and even a healthy snack.

7 Day Meal Plan

You will find a 7 day meal plan listed below. This is just an example of the types of meals you can include in your weekly menus.

Monday

> Breakfast- one serving of "Crusted Bacon Frittata Muffins"
> Lunch-one serving of "Watercress & Spinach Keto Salad"
> Dinner- one serving of "Cheeseburger Bacon Casserole"
> Side dish- "Creamy Cauliflower Mashed Potatoes"
> Dessert (optional)- "Peanut Butter & Coconut Balls" eat as many as you can
>
> Total calories: 1393 (excluding dessert)
>
> Approximate cost: $5.61

Tuesday

- Breakfast- 2 servings "Low Carb Hunger Ending Bacon Frittatas"
- Lunch- 1 serving "Bacon Cheeseburger Casserole"
- Dinner- 1 serving "Salmon Cakes with Herbs"
- Side Dish- 1 serving "Spicy Lemon Roasted Broccoli"
- Dessert (optional)- as many "Peanut Butter & Coconut Balls" that you can eat

Total calories (minus dessert) 1312

Approximate cost: $6.73

Wednesday

- Breakfast- 1 serving "Crusted Bacon Frittata Muffins"
- Lunch- 1 serving of "Watercress & Spinach Keto Salad"
- Dinner- 1 servings "Bacon Cheeseburger Casserole"
- Side Dish- 1 serving of "Creamy Cauliflower Mashed Potatoes"
- Dessert- (optional) - as many "Peanut Butter & Coconut Balls" as you can eat

Total Calories- (minus dessert) - 1393

Approximate cost- $5.61

Thursday

- Breakfast- 1 serving of "Low Carb Hunger Ending Bacon Frittatas"
- Lunch- 1 serving "Bacon Cheeseburger Casserole"
- Dinner- 1 serving "Salmon Cakes with Herbs"
- Side dish- 1 serving- "Lemon Roasted Spicy Broccoli"
- Dessert- "1 Churro Mug Cake"

Total Calories- 1510

Approximate cost- $7.37

Friday

- Breakfast- 1 serving of "Crusted Bacon Frittata Muffins"
- Lunch- 1 serving- "Spinach Watercress Keto Salad"
- Dinner- "Bacon Cheeseburger Casserole"
- Side dish- "Creamy Cauliflower Mashed Potatoes"
- Dessert- "Peanut Butter & Coconut Balls" as many as you can eat

Total Calories 1393

Approximate cost $5.61

Saturday

- Breakfast- 2 servings of "Low-carb Hunger Ending Bacon Frittatas"
- Lunch- 1 servings of "Bacon Cheeseburger Casserole"
- Dinner- 1 serving of "Salmon cakes with herbs"
- Side dish- 1 serving of "Spicy Lemon roasted broccoli"
- Dessert- as many "Peanut Butter & Coconut Balls" as you can eat

Total Calories (excluding dessert) 1312

Approximate cost $6.73

Sunday

- Breakfast- 1 serving of "Crusted Bacon Frittata Muffins"
- Lunch- 1 serving "Watercress & Spinach Keto Salad"
- Dinner- 1 serving of "Cheeseburger Bacon Casserole"
- Side dish- 1 serving "Spicy Lemon roasted broccoli"
- Dessert- as many of the "Peanut Butter & Coconut Balls" you can eat

Total Calories (excluding dessert) 1287

Approximate costs $5.29

Chapter 16
"Recipes for Success"

https://pixabay.com/vectors/recipe-label-icon-symbol-spoon-575434/

The hardest thing about starting a new diet is knowing where to start. This next chapter is going to show you some easy, tasty recipes that go along with your first week's diet plan.

Crusted Bacon Frittata Muffins

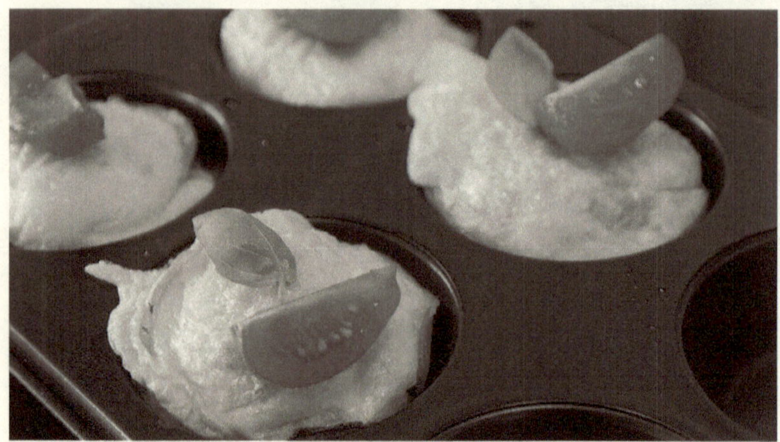

https://pixabay.com/photos/egg-egg-muffin-breakfast-food-ham-682645/

Prep:
18 bacon slices
7 eggs (large)
1 c. shredded cheddar cheese
4 T. whipping cream (heavy)
½ t. black pepper (ground)
½ t. onion powder
½ t. celery salt
½ t. cayenne pepper

Putting it together:
1. preheat oven to 375 Fahrenheit
2. cut bacon slices in half--now place them around the
    outside and bottom of a muffin pan--ensuring to fill in
    any gaps--this should take about 2 slices bacon each
3. Now, place this in the pre-heated oven for about 15--to
    pre-bake them,.
4. While the bacon baskets are baking, stir the eggs, cream,
    and spices together in a bowl.
5. place 1-2 tbsp cheese on the bottom of each bacon cup
6. next scoop about ¼ c. egg mixture into each bacon cup;
    try to keep the egg mixture from leaking out of the cup;
    now put the egg filled bacon cups in the oven for another
    12-15 minutes or until they start to brown.

7. Take out of oven and allow to cool a few minutes before serving.

This recipe makes 7 servings-- you can double the recipe to have enough servings for your entire week's menu plan.

Nutritional information:

18 bacon slices--2102 cal.; 200.04 fat gr.; 6.45 gr. carbs.; 0 gr. fiber; 6.45 gr., net carbs; 63.6 gr. protein

7 eggs (large sized)--500 cal.; 33.28 fat gr.; 2.52 gr. carbs; 0 gr. fiber; 2.52 gr. net carbs; 43.96 gr. protein

1 c. shredded cheddar cheese- 457 cal.; 37.64 fat gr.; 3.79 gr. carbs; 0 gr. fiber; 3.49 net carbs; 25.84 gr. protein

4 T. heavy whipped cream- 204 cal; 21.65 gr. fat; 1.64 gr. carbs; 0.0 fiber; 1.64 net gr. carbs; 1.7 gr. protein

½ t black pepper (ground)- 3 cal.; .01 gr. fat; .74 gr. carbs; .3 gr. fiber; .44 gr. net carbs; .12 gr. protein

½ t. onion powder- 4 cal.; .01 gr. fat; .95 gr. carbs; .2 gr fiber; .75 gr. net carbs.; .12 gr. protein

½ t. celery salt- 0 cal; 0 gr. fat; .0 gr carbs; 0 gr. fibrt; 0 gr. net carts, 0 gr. protein

½ t. cayenne pepper- 3 cal.; .16 fat gr.; .51 gr. carbs; .2 gr. fiber; ;.31 gr. net carbs; .11 gr. protein

Totals: 3273 cal.; 292.82 gr. fat; 16.3 gr. carbs; .7 gr. fiber; 15.6 gr. net carbs; 135.45 gr. protein

Per serving (7): 467.57 cal.; 41.86 gr. fat; 2.33 gr. carbs; .1 gr. fiber; 2.23 gr. net carbs; 19.35 gr. protein

Watercress & Spinach Keto Salad

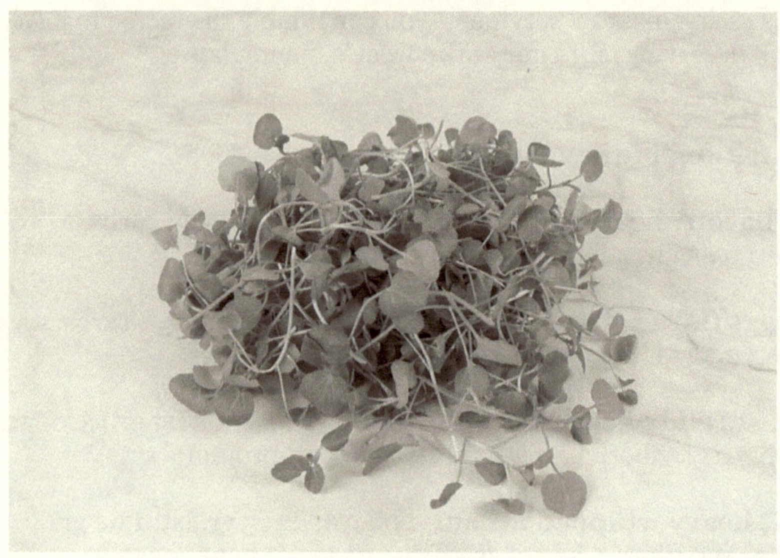

https://pixabay.com/photos/watercress-crazy-la-cresson-4153775/

Ingredients:

1 c. watercress
3 c. baby spinach
1 avocado, medium-sized (sliced)
½ c. Parmesan cheese (shredded)
¼ c. avocado oil
⅛ c. lemon juice
salt and pepper for flavor
1 T. Meditteranean seasoning (optional)

How to put it together:

1. Wash all the greens under cold water; removing stems from the watercress and spinach. Then gently pat it dry.
2. Now put the greens together either on a serving plate or in a big bowl.
3. Peel the avocado and cut in half; remove pit.
4. Slice avocado into thin strips-- set aside

5. Combine lemon juice, avocado oil, Mediterranean seasoning to make dressing; put in a salad oil shaker- shake this together to ensure all ingredients are mixed
6. Now put the shredded Parmesan cheese, avocado, salt/pepper on the top of the spinach/watercress. Gently pour on the dressing and it is ready to eat.

Nutritional Information:

1 cup watercress- 4 calories; 0.03 fat; 0.44 carbs; 0.2 fiber; 0.24 net carbs; 0.78 protein

3 c. baby spinach- 21 calories; 0.35 fat; 3.27 carbs; 0 fiber; 2 net carbs; 2.57 protein

1 med. (136 g) avocado- 227 calories; 20.96 fat; 11.75 carbs; 9.2 fiber; 2.55 net carbs; 2.67 protein

½ c. shredded parmesan cheese- 166 calories; 10.94 fat; 1.36 carbs; 0 fiber; 1.36 net carbs; 15.14 protein

¼ c. avocado oil- 390 calories; 42 fats; 0 carbs; 0 fiber; 0 net carbs; 0 protein

⅛ c. lemon juice- 7 calories; 0.07 fat; 2.1 carbs; 0.1 fiber; 2 net carbs; 0.11 protein

Totals- 815 calories; 74.35 fat; 18.92 carbs; 11.5 fiber; 21.27 net carbs; 21.27 protein

Per servings (4) 203.75 calories; 18.59 fats; 4.73 carbs; 2.88 fiber; 1.85 net carbs; 5.32 protein

Cheeseburger Bacon Casserole

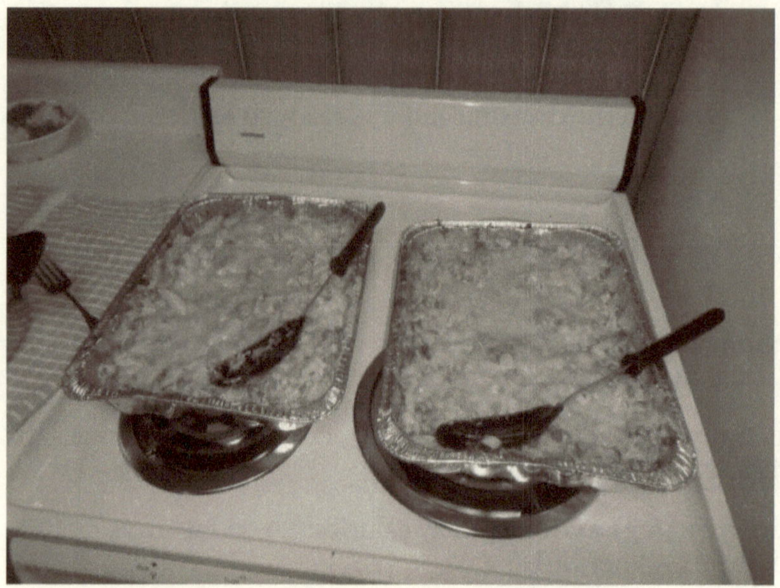

https://images.app.goo.gl/BZx2rY9UpLFEAmfC8

Ingredients

1 pound 80/20 ground beef
3 bacon slices
½ c. almond flour
265 g. riced cauliflower (3 c. chopped)
1 T. *Psyllium Husk Powder*
½ t. garlic powder
½ t. onion powder
2 T. ketchup (low sugar)
1 T. mustard (dijon)
2 T. Mayonaise
3 eggs (large)
4 ounces cheese (cheddar) -- 2 ounces for the inside/2 ounces for the top
salt and pepper for flavoring

Now let's put it together

1. Set your oven to 350 fahrenheit and allow to pre-heat. Put the cauliflower in a food processor and get it to rice texture. Combine all the dry items together

2. Put the ground beef and bacon in the food processor and process that together until it gets crumbly and a bit pasty texture. Cook this over a medium temperature and flavor with salt and pepper.
3. While the meat mixture is cooking, shred the cheese. When meat is finished cooking, put all the elements together in a big bowl and put 2 ounces of the cheddar cheese it.
4. Put the eggs, ketchup, mustard, and mayonnaise into this mixture and mix together really good using a fork or your hands.
5. Next, place in a 9x9 baking dish that has been first lined with waxed paper. Press it gently into the pan and top with the remaining 2 ounces of cheddar cheese.
6. Bake for 25-30 minutes on the top rack of your oven. If you want it extra crispy, you can put in the broiler for 2-3 minutes longer.
7. Let cool for 5-10 minutes outside the oven.
8. Now you can slice it up; garnish with other items-- such as mustard, more low-sugar ketchup, or pickles.

Yield 6 servings. 478 calories each; 35.5 fat grams; 3.6 net carbs, and 32.2 protein grams.

Nutritional Information:

1 lb. ground beef- 1232 calories; 80 fat; 0 carbs; 0 fiber; 0 net carbs; 120 protein

3 slices bacon- 345 calories; 32 fat; 0 carbs; 0 fiber; 0 net carbs; 11 protein

½ c. almond flour- 320 calories; 32 fat; 0 carbs; 0 fiber; 0 net carbs; 11 protein

265 g. riced cauliflower- 66 calories; 0 fat; 14 carbs; 7 fiber; 7 net carbs; 5 protein

1 T. Psyllium Husk- 30 calories; 0 fat; 8 carbs; 7 fiber; 1 net carbs; 0 protein

½ t. garlic powder- 4 calories; 0 fat; 1 carbs; 0 fiber; 1 net carbs; 1 protein

½ t. onion powder- 4 calories; 0 fat; 1 carb; 0 fiber; 1 net carb; 0 protein

salt & pepper to taste- 3 calories; 0 fat; 0 carb; 0 fiber; 0 net carb; 0 protein

2 T. RS Ketchup- 10 calories; 0 fat; 2 carbs; 0 fiber; 2 net carbs; 0 protein

1 T. Dijon mustard- 4 calories; 0 fat; 0 carbs; 0 fiber; 0 net carbs 0 protein

2 T. Mayonnaise- 180 calories; 20 fat; 0 carbs; 0 fiber; 0 net carbs; 0 protein

3 Lg eggs- 210 calories; 15 fat; 1.5 carbs; 0 fiber; 1.5 net carbs; 18 protein

4 oz. cheddar cheese- 460 calories; 38 fats; 0 carbs; 0 fiber; 2 net carbs; 27 protein

Totals- 286 calories; 213 fats; 41.5 carbs; 20 fiber; 21.5 net carbs; 193 protein

per serving (6)- 478 calories; 35.5 fats; 6.9 carbs; 3.3 fiber; 3.6 net carbs; 32.2 protein

Creamy Cauliflower Mashed Potatoes

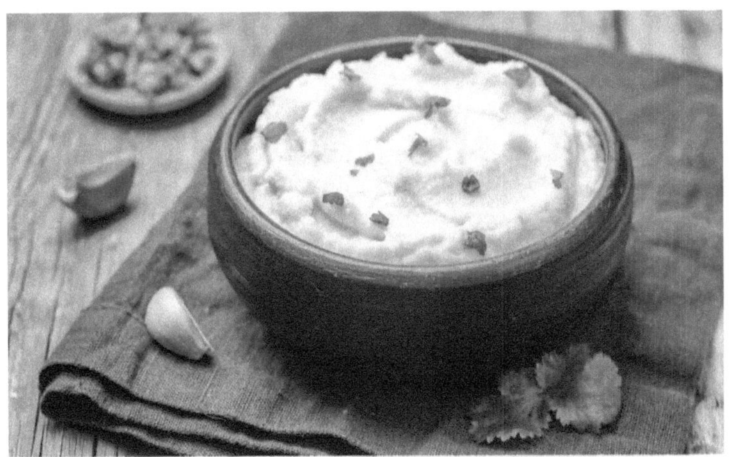

https://images.app.goo.gl/PcfToRGaacDysiFm9

Ingredients

10 oz riced cauliflower (refrigerated)
¼ c. sour cream
3 T. whipping cream (heavy)
3 T. butter
4 T. Parmesan cheese
¼ t. garlic powder
2 T. chives (chopped)
flavored with salt and pepper

Let's put it together:

1. First, take the cauliflower you have already riced out of the refrigerator and measure out 10 ounces.
2. Put it in a microwave safe container, cover with a paper towel, cook it for 5 minutes. **if you prefer, you can steam or roast the cauliflower.
3. Cauliflower should be soft yet firm
4. Now stir the remaining ingredients into the cauliflower
5. Using the immersion setting on a blender; blend these ingredients together completely; add one tablespoon of chives to this mixture
6. Next, top with the remaining chives and serve!

This recipe yields 3 servings: 243.67 calories; 22.74 fat grams; 4.53 net carbs; 5.7 protein grams.

Nutritional Information:

10 ounces cauliflower, riced 71 calories; 0.79 fat grams; 14.07 carbs; 5.7 fiber; 8.37 net carbs; 6.16 protein

¼ cup sour cream 114 calories; 11.13 fats; 2.66 carbs; 0 fiber; 2.66 net carbs; 1.4 protein

3 tablespoons heavy whipping cream
153 calories; 16.24 fat grams; 1.23 carbs; 0 fiber; 1.23 net carbs; 1.28 protein

3 tablespoons butter 305 calories; 34.55 fats; 0.03 carbs; 0 fiber; 0.03 net carbs; 0.36 protein

4 tablespoons Parmesan cheese83 calories; 5.47 fats; 0.68 carbs; 0 fiber; 0.68 net carbs; 7.57 protein

¼ teaspoon garlic powder 3 calories; 0.01 fats; 0.56 carbs; 0.1 fiber; 0.46 net carbs; 0.13 protein

2 tablespoons chopped chives 2 calories; 0.04 fats; .26 carbs; 0.1 fiber; 0.16 net carbs; .2 protein

Totals 731 calories; 68.23 fats; 19.49 carbs; 5.9 fiber; 13.59 net carbs; 17.1 protein

Per Serving 243.67 calories; 22.74 fats; 6.5 carbs; 1.97 fiber; 4.53 net carbs; 5.7 protein

Peanut Butter & Coconut Balls

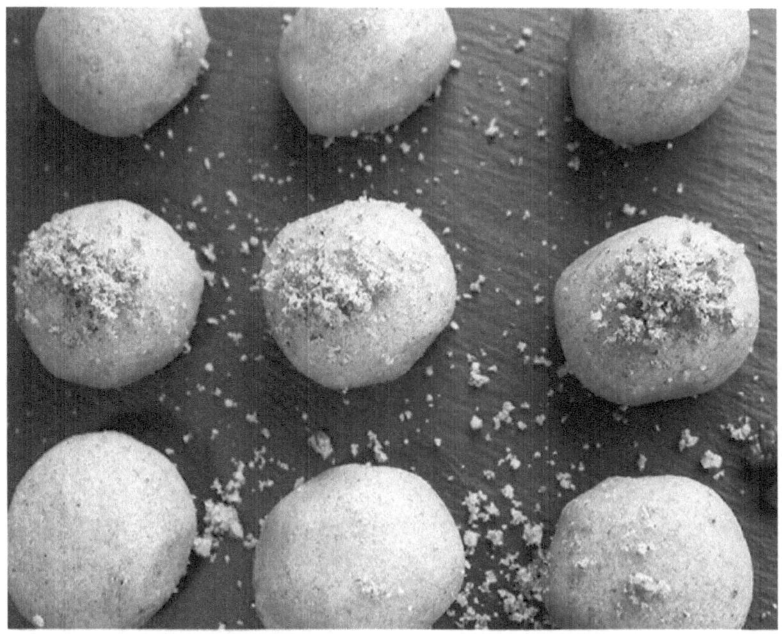

https://images.app.goo.gl/EadyHD8oG1K9VDmf8

Ingredients

3 T. peanut butter (creamy style)
3. unsweetened cocoa powder
2.5 t. erythritol (powered)
2 t. almond flour
½ c. unsweetened coconut (shredded)

Let's put it all together:

1. Put the peanut butter, cocoa powder, erythritol, and flour in a bowl and mix it together
2. Freeze this mixture for 1 hour
3. Spoon out this mixture using a melon baller or small spoon
4. Drop balls into shredded coconut; roll around in the coconut and form into a ball with your hands;
5. Refrigerate overnight

This recipe nets 15 balls; each ball has 35.13 calories; 3.19 fats; 0.92 net carbs; 0.98 protein

Nutritional Information:

3 tablespoons creamy peanut butter 287 calories; 24.65 fats; 10.71 carbs; 2.4 fiber; 8.31 net carbs; 10.66 protein

3 teaspoons unsweetened cocoa powder 12 calories; 0.74 fats; 3.13 carbs; 2 grams fiber; 1.13 net carbs; 1.06 protein

2 ½ teaspoons powdered erythritol 0 calories; 0 fats; 0 carbs; 0 fiber; 0 net carbs; 0 protein

2 teaspoons of almond flour 28 calories; 2.46 fats; 0.82 carbs; 0.5 fiber; 0.32 net carbs; 0.98 protein

½ cup unsweetened coconut flakes 200 calories; 20 fats; 8 carbs; 4 fiber; 4 net carbs; 2 protein

Totals 527 calories; 47.85 fats; 22.66 carbs; 8.9 fiber; 13.76 net carbs; 14.7 protein;

Per serving 25.13 calories; 3.19 fats; 1.51 carbs; 0.59 fiber; 0.92 net carbs; 0.98 protein

Low Carb Hunger Ending Frittata Bars

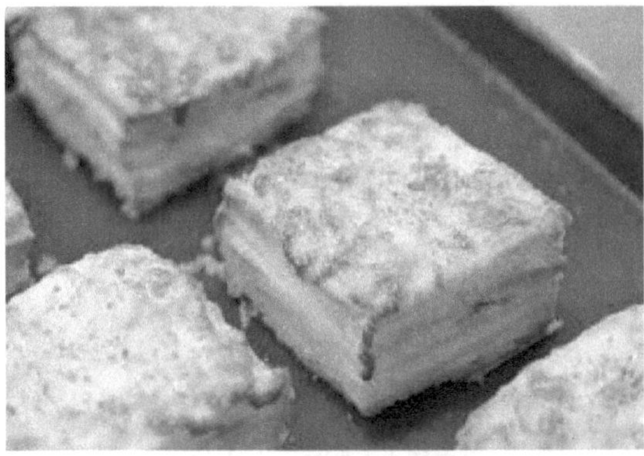

https://images.app.goo.gl/EzNqB3wTCrWZNwNh7

Elements you will need:

8 eggs (large)
½ c. "half-n- half" creamer
6 oz bacon-- cooked & cut up in small pieces
½ c. cheese (cheddar)
1 T. real butter
2 t. parsley (dried)
½ t. pepper (black)
¼ t. salt
sauteed spinach; minced broccoli; of a bit of onion (optional ingredients)

Let's get it together:

1. First step, need to get your oven heated to a toasty 375 degrees fahrenheit. Be sure to have the bacon already fried, chopped, and ready!
2. Next step--crack open the eggs and mix ½ n ½ in a mixing bowl.
3. Stir this mixture together well until eggs are nearly scrambled--you will still want some egg white streaks to show
4. Slowly stir in bacon, cheese, dried parsley, pepper and salt.

5. Prepare a muffin pan by greasing it with butter--for about 8 muffins
6. Fill each muffin cup ¾ full of this egg mixture
7. Bake 15-18 minutes in the preheated oven; till puffy and golden brown
8. Take out and let sit for a minute to cool
9. Serve and enjoy!

Yields 8 servings
Each serving has 248.63 calories; 19.33 fat grams; 1.66 net carb grams; 16.03 net protein grams.

Nutritional Information:
8 lg. eggs- 572 calories; 38.04 fat; 2.88 carbs; 0 fiber; 2.88 net carbs; 50.24 protein

½ c. half-n-half- 149 calories; 12.57 fat; 5.72 carbs; 0 fiber; 5.72 net carbs; 3.79 protein

6 oz. bacon- 932 calories; 73.56 fat; 2.29 carbs; 0 fiber; 2.29 net carbs; 60.74 protein

½ c. cheddar cheese- 228 calories; 18.82 fat; 1.75 carbs; 0 fiber; 1.75 net carbs; 12.92 protein

1 T. butter- 102 calories; 11.52 fat; 0.01 carbs; 0 fiber; 0.01 net carbs; 0.12 protein

2 t. dried parsley- 3 calories; 0.05 fat; 0.51 carbs; 0.3 fiber; 0.21 net carbs; 0.27 protein

½ t. pepper- 3 calories; 0.04 fat; 0.74 carbs; 0.3 fiber; 0.44 net carbs; 0.12 protein

Total- 1989 calories; 154.6 fat; 13.9 carbs; 0.6 fiber; 13.3 net carbs; 128.2 protein

Per serving- 248.63 calories; 19.33 fat; 1.74 carbs; 0.08 fiber; 1.66 net carbs; 16.03 protein

Salmon Cakes with Herbs

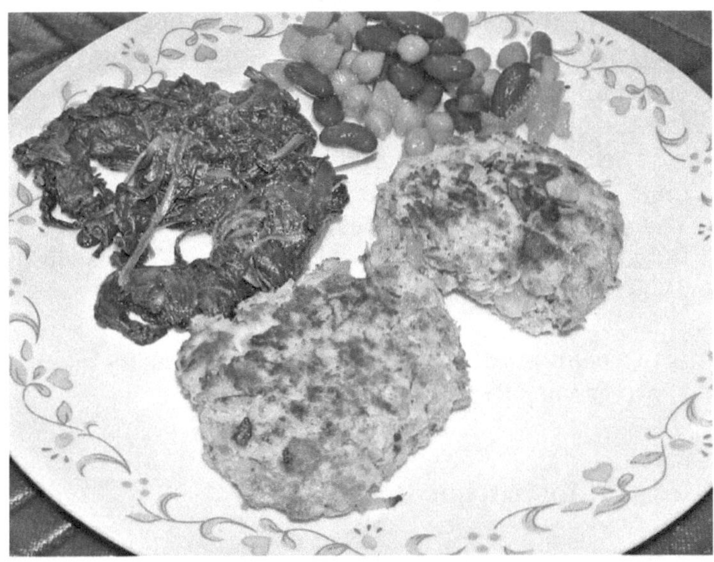

https://pixabay.com/photos/spinach-bean-salad-salmon-cakes-655479/

What you will need:

2- 14.57 oz. cans of pink salmon
2 T. chopped chives (fresh)
1/4 c. dill (fresh, chopped)
¼ c. grated Parmesan cheese
4 oz. crushed pork rinds
2 eggs (large)
1 t. lemon peel
salt/pepper for flavoring
½ c. almond flour
2 T. olive oil

Now let's put it together:

1. Open up both cans salmon--drain the juices out and empty cans into a large bowl
2. Now add in the chives, dill, cheese, pork rinds, eggs, lemon peel, salt/pepper

3. Stir this all up really well--
4. Then form about 10 balls out of this mixture
5. Pour the flour on a plate; place each ball on the plate and roll in the flour
6. Then take the palm of your hand and gently flatten out each ball
7. Put the olive oil in a skillet; heat the oil up
8. Place each salmon cake in the pan and cook a few minutes on each side until browned lightly and done
9. You can serve the salmon cakes with some lemon and a little bit of homemade tartar sauce (recipe below) and a plate of steamed veggies.

A serving is 2 salmon cakes which has 418 calories; 25 fat grams; 2.63 net carb grams; 46 grams of protein.

Nutritional Information

2 (14.75 oz) cans of pink salmon- 1072.73 calories; 40.23 fat; 0 carbs; 0 fiber; 0 net carbs; 174.32 protein

2 T. chopped fresh chives- 1.8 calories; 0.04 fat; 0.26 carbs; 0.15 fiber; 0.11 net carbs; 0.2 protein

¼ c. chopped fresh dill- 31.37 calories; 0.54 fat; 6.92 carbs; 1.69 fiber; 5.23 net carbs; 2.48 protein

¼ c. grated Parmesan Cheese- 120 calories; 8 fats; 2 carbs; 1 fiber; 1 net carbs; 10 protein

4 oz pork rinds (crushed)- 160 calories; 10 fats; 0 carbs; 0 fiber; 0 net carbs; 16 protein

2 Large eggs- 143 calories; 9.31 fats; 0.72 carbs; 0 fiber; 12.56 protein

1 teaspoon zest of a lemon- 1 calorie; 0 fat; 0.3 carbs; 0.2 fiber; 0.1 net carbs; 0 protein

salt & pepper- 0 calorie; 0 fat; 0 carbs; 0 fiber; 0 net carbs; 0 protein

½ c. almond flour- 320 calories; 28 fat; 12 carbs; 6 fiber; 6 net carbs; 12 protein

2 T. olive oil- 238.68 calories; 27 fats; 0 carbs; 0 fiber; 0 net carbs; 0 protein

Totals- 2088.58 calories; 123.32 fat; 22.2 carbs; 9.04 fiber; 13.16 net carbs; 227.56 protein

Per serving (5)- 417.72 calories; 24.66 fat; 4,44 carbs; 1,81 fiber; 2.63 net carbs; 4.51 protein

Homemade Tartar Sauce

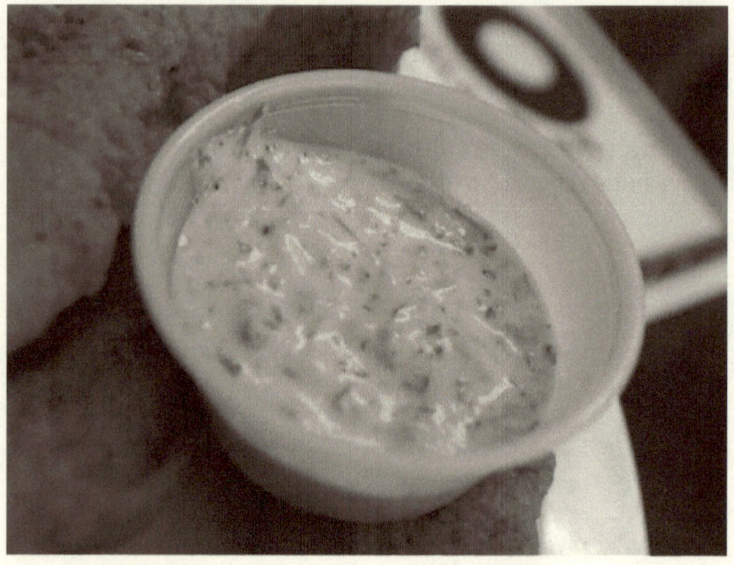

https://images.app.goo.gl/dwDAng6KfhuCCa5V9

Ingredients:

½ c. mayo
1 T. dill pickles-diced
1 t. lemon juice
1 t. green onion (finely diced)
½ t. dill weed

Mix it up:

Add all the above ingredients into a small bowl and mix up completely. Serve with your Salmon cakes!

A serving of tartar sauce is about 1 Tablespoon: 130.48 calories; 14.91 fat grams; 0.32 net carb grams; 0.6 protein grams

Nutritional Information:

½ cup mayonnaise- 104.08 calories; 119.2 fat; 1.84 carbs; 0 fiber; 1.84 net carbs; 4.64 protein

1 tablespoon diced dill pickle- 1 calorie; 0.03 fat; 0.21 carbs; 0.11 nets carbs; 0.04 protein

1 teaspoon lemon juice- 1 calorie; 0.01 fat; 0.34 carbs; 0 fiber; 0.34 net carbs; 0.02 protein

1 teaspoon finely diced green onion- 0 calories; 0 fat; 0.06 carbs; 0 fiber; 0.06 net carbs; 0.01 protein

½ teaspoon of dill weed- 1 calorie; 0.0 fat; 0.025 carbs; 0.1 fiber; 0.18 net carbs; 0.1 protein

Totals- 1043.8 calories; 119.26 fat; 2.7 carbs; 0.2 fiber; 2.53 net carbs; .26 protein

Per servings (8)- 130.48 calories; 14.91 fat; 0.34 carbs; 0.03 fiber; 0.32 net carbs; 0.06 protein

Spicy Lemon Roasted Broccoli

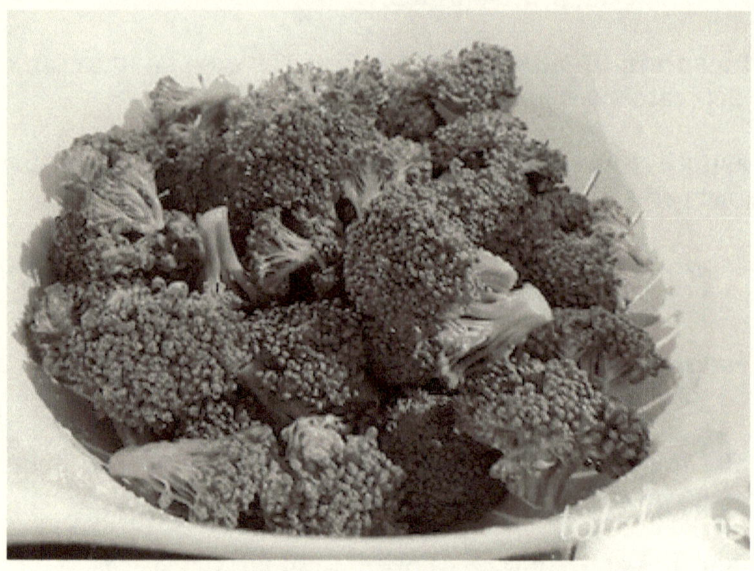

https://images.app.goo.gl/tLXHCtM3TCfvWZPq9

What you will need:

1-½ lbs. of broccoli (florets)
⅓ c. parmesan cheese
¼ c. olive oil
2 T. basil (fresh & chopped)
3 t. garlic (minced)
½ to ¾ t. kosher salt
½ t. red chili flakes
½ t. lemon juice & zest

Now let's put it all together

1. Prepare your oven by preheating it to a toasty 425 degrees fahrenheit. Cover a cooking sheet with waxed paper first, then arrange the broccoli florets in one layer on the sheet.
2. Next you need to season the broccoli with some olive oil, chopped fresh basil, minced garlic, kosher salt, red chili flakes, lemon juice and zest.
3. Sprinkle the Parmesan cheese all over the top. Place in the oven for 20-25 minutes

4. Take out of oven and enjoy!

There are six servings total with 1 serving being about 138.17 calories; 10.77 fat grams; 5.24 net carb grams; 4.83 protein grams.

Nutritional Information:

1-½ pound broccoli florets- 216 calories; 2.38 fats; 42.16 carbs; 16.5 fiber; 25.66 net carbs; 17.91 protein

⅓ cup shredded parmesan- 111 carbs; 7.91 fat; 0.91 carbs; 0 fiber; 0.91 net carbs; 10.09 protein

⅓ cup olive oil- 477 calories; 54 fats; 0 carb; 0 fiber; 0 net carbs; 0 protein

2 Tablespoon fresh chopped basil- 1 calories; 0.03 fat; 0.14 carbs; 0.1 fiber; 0.04 net carbs; 0.17 protein

3 teaspoons minced garlic- 13 calories; 0.04 fat; 2.78 carbs; 0.2 fiber; 2.58 net carbs; 0.53 protein

½ teaspoon red chili flakes- 3 calories; 0.16 fat; 0.51 carbs; .2 fiber; 0.31 net carbs; 0.11 protein

½ teaspoon zest of a lemon- 8 calories; 0.08 fat; 2.62 carbs; 0.7 fiber; 1.92 net carbs; 0.17 protein

Totals- 829 calories; 64.6 fat; 49.12 carbs; 17.7 fiber; 31.42 net carbs; 28.98 protein

per servings (6)- 138.17 calories; 10.77 fat; 8.19 carbs; 2.95 fiber; 5.24 net carbs; 4.83 protein

Conclusion

We sincerely hope that "Keto Way of Life- Ketogenic Plans for a Healthier Life" has been an excellent source of information and resources for starting and maintaining a Keto lifestyle.

Thank you again for downloading this book!

We hope this book was able to help you to understand more completely what the "Keto Way of Life- Ketogenic Plans for A Healthier Life" is all about and how it can change your life for the better.

Finally, if you enjoyed the Keto Lifestyle, please take the time to share your thoughts and post a review on Amazon. It'd be greatly appreciated!

Thank you and good luck!

About the Authors

Teresa Fikes

Teresa has been living the Keto Lifestyle and reaping the rewards. After only a couple of months, lost 20 lbs. Then continued on to lose weight and maintain a healthy lifestyle.

After suffering the pain of fatty liver disease and high sugar levels, if was time for a change. After only 6 months of living the Keto Lifestyle all test came back with normal levels. She experience more energy, and all around better health.

Teresa has over 40 years of homesteading experience. She loves anything to do with living off the land on and off the grid. She believes in being self-sufficient. She raises her own foods, medicines, and crafts. Also, she is a really big fan of clean eating and pressure cooker recipes, as you can see within many of her different Homesteading series of books and e-books. Teresa specializes in and is a fan of Homesteading Skills which include raising meat rabbits, chickens, goats, hogs, cows, horses, ducks, poultry, and dogs, as well has all kinds of fruits, vegetables, and herbs. She collects wild foods and hunts for what she doesn't raise on her small farm.

Teresa's homesteading series includes many book topics such as Home Brewing, slow cooker, clean eating, instant pot, crockpot, electric pressure cooker recipes, baking recipes, preserving, foraging, planting, building, and the list goes on.

Having a well-stocked pantry of easy to open and serve jars of food is essential for a busy family, whether farming, survival prepping, or just the normal city dweller. Follow Teresa to discover more about Homesteading Life Skills.

Read more of Teresa's book on Amazon Author Page

Georgann R. Fohner

Georgann has been writing short stories and poetry for several years. She won a Golden Poetry award for a poem *"Where is Our Logic and Sense of Reason"* that she wrote when she was younger.

This is Georgann's 5th eBook and you can find them all at <u>Amazon.com</u>.

Georgann has worked for 30 years in the field of Human Services. She loves helping others learn how to live a self-sufficient and healthy life. She has a Master's Degree in Criminal Justice and also works as a freelance writer, writing blogs and content for articles.

Georgann is married and has one son, 24 years old. Her son is attending college and hopes to go into a field in which he, too, can help people to live better lives.

**Look for many more eBooks in the near future that Georgann and Teresa will be writing together. From the paranormal to how to cook, eat, and live a healthier lifestyle.

Thank you!

www.ingramcontent.com/pod-product-compliance
Lightning Source LLC
Chambersburg PA
CBHW051219250726
48655CB00006B/2491